THE TIBETAN
BOOK OF HEALING

THE TIBETAN
BOOK OF HEALING

by Dr. Lopsang Rapgay, Ph.D.

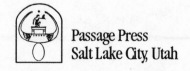
Passage Press
Salt Lake City, Utah

DISCLAIMER

This book is a reference work not intended to treat, diagnose or prescribe. The information contained herein is in no way to be considered as a substitute for consultation with a duly licensed health-care professional.

Passage Press is a division of Morson Publishing
Morson Publishing
P.O. Box 21713
Salt Lake City, Utah 84121-0713

Published 1997

Printed in the United States of America

Cover design by Reed L. Perkins

Library of Congress Catalog Card Number: 96-72086
ISBN 1-878423-21-5

This book is dedicated to my root teacher the late Kyabche Trichang Rimpoche, junior tutor to His Holiness the Dalai Lama, and my late father Karma Wangchuk Sherpa

CONTENTS

ACKNOWLEDGMENTS

I would like to thank Yola Jurzykoski of the Shen Foundation, San Francisco, for the initial grant to write this book; also Linda Merle, Kevin Lagden and Michael Connelly for their editing and suggestions.

FOREWORD
By David Frawley, O.M.D.

Tibetan medicine is an ancient, systematic and integral system of mind-body medicine containing a wealth of knowledge and experience along with many practical methods of health improvement. It deserves more attention in the modern world now that we are focusing on traditional and alternative systems to help deal with the inadequacies of present drug-based medicine.

Tibetan medicine is primarily a form of Ayurveda, which was not only the traditional natural healing system of India but through history influenced surrounding cultures from Greece to China. Ayurveda is the basis of Indian Buddhist medicine, and was transmitted along with Buddhism to Tibet. Tibetan medicine, it should be noted, does combine important aspects of Chinese medicine as well, but Ayurveda constitutes the main portion of its theory, practice and herbal preparations. For this reason Tibetan medicine could well be called "Tibetan Ayurveda" or "Buddhist Ayurveda." However while there are a number of popular books on Ayurveda available in the West today, there has been little comparable on Tibetan medicine, or showing the links between the two.

The Buddhist contribution to Ayurvedic medicine is considerable. With its emphasis on compassion Buddhist kings and teachers in India promoted Ayurvedic hospitals and Ayurvedic learning to help alleviate the suffering of living beings. Ayurveda, as its name indicates, grew out of a Vedic (Hindu) basis, through the work of the Vedic seers, and employs a Vedic terminology. However many Buddhists helped develop it, particularly during its later periods. Ayurvedic practices are mentioned in Buddhist literature as current during the time of Buddha himself.

There are three main classics of Ayurveda: *Caraka Samhita* of Caraka, *Susruta Samhita* of Susruta, and *Astanga Hrdaya* of Vagbhatta. *Caraka Samhita* is the oldest of the three, but *Susruta* is also very old, and both in their earlier materials reflect the late Vedic era before Buddha (500 B.C.). Vagbhatta, whose work contains the material of Caraka and Susruta condensed in verse form, was a Buddhist who lived in Sind (the lower Indus region) around 500 A.D. The present version of *Susruta Samhita* is attributed to a redaction done by the famous Buddhist Siddha Nagarjuna, who flourished in South India about two thousand years ago, and is perhaps the most famous figure in northern (Mahayana) Buddhism after Buddha. Nagarjuna was most noted for introducing alchemical formulations into Ayurveda and is still honored in South India today for this work. Hence one of the three great classics of Ayurveda one comes from a Buddhist and another has been edited by a great Buddhist sage. Tibetan medical practitioners still today commonly study Vagbhatta, but some also refer to Caraka and Susruta.

The Buddhist contribution to Ayurveda is perhaps greatest in the field of psychology, in which Buddhism adds its unique approach to the mind. Buddhism is a highly psychological approach to spirituality and has great depth in this regard. *The Tibetan Book of Healing* shows the Buddhist psychological approach to healing and how it interfaces with Ayurveda whose very concept of the biological humors has an inherent psychological component.

Tibetan Buddhism is primarily of the Tantric variety which, with its emphasis on yogic practices, including special methods of rejuvenation and immortality, has always been linked with Ayurveda. Tantra and Ayurveda have long been sister sciences in both Hindu and Buddhist traditions and together contain a system for understanding the entire process of spiritual unfoldment, including the physiological changes that it brings.

Tibetan medicine bases itself on the three Ayurvedic constitutional types of Vata (air), Pitta (fire) and Kapha (water), called Lung, Tripa and Bagan in Tibetan. It provides another slant on the Ayurvedic constitutional approach based upon these three types, which Dr. Rapgay calls "Tibetan constitutional typology." Those who know their Ayurvedic type will benefit from looking at it from a Tibetan perspective as well.

The Tibetan Book of Healing introduces the system of Tibetan medicine in both a comprehensive and practical manner, including theory, diagnosis and treatment. The author, Dr. Lobsang Rapgay, is one of the foremost Tibetan doctors in the world today, and is also a psychologist. He has practiced clinical Ayurvedic methods like Pancha Karma as well and introduces a Tibetan approach to it.

His book is welcome in several ways. First it is an explication of Tibetan medicine by a trained Tibetan doctor working in the United States. So far Tibetan medicine has largely been dealt with only on an academic level, and its presentations have often referred to Tibetan life-style concerns which can be very different than those in the West today. Second the book serves as a bridge to link Tibetan medicine with Ayurveda, which allows Ayurvedic students to add the Tibetan perspective to their approach. Third and above all, it contains many helpful practices, going into diet, herbs, and meditation and providing a number of methods and techniques to follow for self-healing purposes.

The book introduces many of the spiritual approaches of Buddhist medicine, including ways of managing emotions and developing compassion. It contains some material on astrology, which is more Chinese in origin, as well. Though small it contains a wealth of information that will make the book a constant companion for those really seeking to improve their state of well-being.

Dr. David Frawley, O.M.D.
Santa Fe New Mexico
April 1995

David Frawley is author of *Ayurvedic Healing, Yoga of Herbs, Tantric Yoga and the Wisdom Goddesses: Spiritual Secrets of Ayurveda*, etc.

1
HEALTH
AND WELLNESS

INTRODUCTION

When we think about our health, we are actually accustomed to thinking in terms of disease. We learn about health from observing what doctors do or say when we are sick. When we feel fine, we rarely think about our health or what we need to do to maintain it. We wait for debilitating symptoms to arise before we realize something must be done.

Nowadays we are learning much more about the importance of taking good care of ourselves. Proper nutrition and adequate exercise are concepts of wellness which are now widely recognized. Unfortunately, however, activities such as jogging, aerobics, or dieting can easily be overdone at the expense of other components of health.

Holistic health, as taught in the Tibetan tradition, does not begin with the idea of disease, nor does it end with the arbitrary adoption of some new exercise program or diet scheme. Holistic health comes from knowing how to assess our body's needs, measure our body's innate strengths and capacities, and, on that basis, to develop for ourselves an appropriate and realistic health plan.

To accomplish this, we must take into account not only our physical condition, but our mental condition as well. The mental factors which determine our attitude toward life, the way we deal with our physical and social surroundings, etc., significantly influence our health. Depressive episodes may be initiated by denying our spiritual needs, resisting psycho-social adjustments or sticking to a deficient diet. Symptoms such as fatigue, lethargy, sluggish digestion and a host of other ills can be relieved by learning what holistic health truly means.

We can now begin to see how any attempt to standardize health and wellness is a difficult process, since it involves so many components unique to each person and his or her environment. The World Health Organization has defined health as "a state of complete physical, mental and social well-being, and not the mere absence of disease or infirmity." Many people in the field of health feel that this definition is so broad that it borders on the meaningless and impractical. Yet it contains the essential concepts that govern genuine holistic health. It takes into account not only the condition of your body but also the state of your mind. How we think, perceive and conceptualize influences our health, perhaps more than anything else. These mental factors determine the attitudes we have about life, the way we deal with our physical and social surroundings and how we interact with others. Health and wellness, therefore, must encompass all of these and be presented in a manner that we can relate to and readily apply. We must learn to recognize the role played by physical, psychological, emotional, social, spiritual and environmental factors in contributing to the overall quality of our lives. There are several ways that we can begin to care for ourselves in a truly holistic fashion. Tibetan medical and Buddhist psychological guidelines have been used for centuries by spiritual masters and practitioners to approach life in a healthy and balanced manner. In our own lives, such guidelines are essential in view of the rate at which we are constantly bombarded with information about how we should care for ourselves.

How do we know which diet is most appropriate, which exercises are most suitable, or whether meditation and relaxation will be beneficial for us? In our already busy and stressful lives, it is difficult to find the time and energy to simultaneously practice all of these health-promoting activities. Which ones should we choose and how should we begin?

Tibetan Buddhist physicians suggest completing a constitutional typology test which is devised to help you find out about your body — how it responds to changes in psychological and physical needs, its potential to meet those needs, and its relationship to climate and environment. By evaluating your priorities and capacities and how you fulfill them in terms of your health, you can obtain a comprehensive understanding of your weaknesses and strengths.

Traditionally, such a test is conducted in two stages. The first consists of an extensive and formal medical procedure that requires the client to undergo a two-week dietary and behavioral regimen. During the second stage of the test, the physician analyzes the client's physical and psychological profile by reading the pulse, examining the urine, inspecting the body and asking questions. In India and Tibet, where most patients were aware of their personality profiles, literacy levels were low, and social and cultural factors were restrictive, this stage of the test was always done with the help of a physician through formal medical procedure. Now, however, a simplified test has been devised based on the medical personality test traditionally administered by the physician. It can be conducted by the client himself or herself, using the score sheet provided to determine his or her own profile. In Chapter 3, a shortened version of this self-administered medical-psychological test is presented. Readers should use it together with the other material in this book to determine their overall health plans.

There are enormous advantages to using the Tibetan constitutional typology test (or any good self-evaluation test or system, for that matter). It allows you to know yourself, examine yourself, and, based on what you discover, to model your own health plan. Why you deal with anger differently than someone else, or why your body type is what it is, are important considerations. A critical evaluation of yourself is necessary because health is not something achieved at a specific time, like getting a college degree. Rather, it is an ongoing process, a way of life.

There will be a whole range of questions running through your mind when you begin thinking about holistic health. The most common problem for people who wish to make changes in their health is: not knowing where to start. Should I modify my diet, exercise my body by jogging or doing aerobics, or try to motivate myself by improving my work habits or personal relationships? Is it possible to work with all of these methods simultaneously, or should I work with them one at a time? And what about occasionally experiencing fatigue, despondency or disinterest in work or play, or failing to organize my time properly or use my potential fruitfully? Are these separate problems, outside the scope of a general health plan, or will they disappear when I put my health plan in motion? All of these questions come to mind.

Another common problem is not knowing when or how to start a health plan. Should I start on a health plan immediately, or should I first prepare myself for such a major change by seeking the counsel of a health expert or by initiating a detoxifying therapy such as colonics? Moreover, when developing a health plan, should I begin immediately *on my own*, without any medical check-ups or tests? Evaluating yourself — your body weight, your history of health, whether you are deficient in any nutrients or lack regular exercise — is crucial before beginning a health program. To jump in immediately, even under conditions such as those in a special health clinic, without first giving serious consideration to these questions, will prove unproductive and dangerous.

Just as perplexing as the problems mentioned above is the question of how to evaluate the effectiveness of current health plans. How do you know, for instance, if a change to a vegetarian or macrobiotic diet, or to a more physically active lifestyle, is appropriate for you? To what degree can such a plan answer your health needs? Is therapy that involves assertive and motivational development sufficient to correct your sense of disinterest in your work or your experiences of fatigue and procrastination? Must you include changes in nutrition, behavior (such as getting additional exercise and relaxation), and psychology? Is a weight-loss program alone sufficient to ensure your ability to control your weight in the future?

You may decide to see a health advisor such as a stress and relaxation specialist, nutritionist, herbalist, acupuncturist, Indian doctor or Tibetan physician. But do you need to consult several such healers before you implement a health plan? If a

Chinese physician explains that you have a congenitally weak liver and that your health plan should revolve around stimulating the liver by diet, exercise, herbs, and meditative and energy-channeling exercises, should you consider this an explanation of your present state of health? Would it not be prudent to consider other possible components of your health, such as low self-esteem and personality problems, as well as behavioral ones? Whether trained in a Western or Eastern tradition, the specialist you go to uses a particular medical model. He or she will look at your health priorities from a particular point of view (which may or may not encompass all your disorders). For instance, the Chinese physician in the example given above may apply acupuncture based on his diagnosis of a weak liver. But if you were to go to a nutritionist, the recommended treatment might be nutritional supplements to deal with a thyroid or yeast condition. Similarly, a Tibetan physician trained solely in Tibetan medicine might arrive at a diagnosis very much like that of the Chinese physician, but might recommend herbal stimulants and dietary changes rather than acupuncture. So you see, since there is no universal model by which to measure and evaluate *all* your health needs, most health practitioners will make their recommendations based on what they find through their own particular diagnostic procedures. Of course, depending on the skill of the healer, your health needs may be met satisfactorily. There are many fine, skilled natural healers, but, unfortunately, not enough. We must remember that it is not entirely the fault of the examining healers when our condition fails to improve. In fact, each of them may be correct in his or her own diagnosis. The liver may be weak, as the Chinese and Tibetan healers say; or, as the nutritionist maintains, there may be a yeast infection. The point, however, is that even though these diagnostic procedures may be correct in themselves, they may fail to recognize symptoms of a larger problem that might take a little more skill and effort to unfold. The client will improve during the course of the treatment of the liver *chi* or yeast infection, but it is also likely that the condition will return as soon as the treatment is terminated. An evaluation system that not only determines the levels of stress and tension or muscle and metabolic function but also explains the constitutional typology of the client is imperative in order to enable the client and healer to jointly address the complaint.

This is not to say that the Tibetan or Indian tradition of constitutional and personality testing is the best model and should be used by all. On the contrary, what is needed is an expanded model that will not only deal with the complaint but also the person — the whole person who, for the time being, suffers from the complaint.

HOW HEALTHY ARE WE?

Like the quality of life, health is variable, and to ensure uniform health in any society is perhaps impossible. Disease and illness are basic facts of life and vary from society to society. Simply taking care of yourself and your needs alone cannot ensure you optimal health. A number of other factors, many of them out of your control, contribute to your health. The economic status, literacy rate, social and cultural beliefs, and availability of technically trained personnel in a community all combine to shape the health of the individual in that society. You might be doing everything that is good for your health — eating the right food, exercising regularly, and even thinking and working in a positive way — but your health is still severely affected by your environment, the sanitation and health of your neighbors and people you work with, etc.... Moreover, unless you have good medical facilities that will allow you to get regular check-ups, how are you to really know your actual health condition?

Therefore, in determining how healthy you are, you must consider a number of factors. Your physician might find that you are perfectly normal, but that finding cannot ensure your health for any length of time unless you educate yourself in self-care. You might be absolutely healthy this week, but there is no guarantee that you will be fine next week. You might pick up a bacterial infection while eating at a restaurant, or catch a virus that is going around town. When we think about our health, we have to think in terms of the variable and changing nature of our health, ourselves and our environment.

No doctor can ensure perfect health for anyone, nor can anything we do for ourselves keep us free from disease. In addition to constantly working with our health, we must be aware of the threats beyond our control which do exist. This does not mean that we should become too contemplative about the whole issue and look at life and health from a fatalistic point of view. The point which must be understood is that paradoxes in life have to be dealt with and appreciated rather than avoided and denied. When we learn to live in a state that is balanced between assurance and apprehension, we will be able to appreciate more deeply the purpose and nature of life. By becoming aware of all the facets of human existence, we can better cope with the limitations imposed upon us, and at the same time find the motivation and sense of responsibility needed to get on with life in a meaningful manner.

Such an understanding will allow us to deal with tension, worry, and frustration, and to modify our living habits in a healthy fashion. Many of life's problems cannot necessarily be solved. Therefore, we should not *expect* to solve them, either physically or psychologically. An ability to objectively analyze problems with what Buddhists call "a mind of positive detachment" makes life much easier for us. You can become worried and tense when you lose your job or fail to achieve an objective — or you can practice detachment. That is to say, after first evaluating a failure and then contemplating it constructively, detach yourself for a time from any repetitive thoughts about the failure.

Health and wellness can no longer be defined as *merely* removing physical and psychological dysfunction or sticking to dietary or behavioral recommendations made by a physician. It is equally important to have values, a sense of responsibility to yourself, and a deep appreciation for being human. In the *Four Tantras*, the fundamental canon of Tibetan medicine, health and wellness are defined by the following factors:

• Freedom from serious psychological and physical disease

• Adherence to a health plan based on your personality, your body type and needs, and your capacity to fulfill and meet those needs

• An understanding of the changing and impermanent nature of life and, within that understanding, the awareness of a purpose in life

• Acceptance of the stress and change found in relationships, the environment, the seasons and the aging process

• A sense of moral responsibility and a willingness to learn and grow

• A feeling of positive accomplishment, contentment, and appreciation for being human

These characteristics clearly indicate that health is not something that can be instantly obtained. It is an ongoing process, a part of living. Yet awareness of health does not mean that you are constantly pondering everything you eat, think and do. It does not mean that you become a rigid robot who always behaves and thinks on the basis of others' recommendations. Rules and regulations that form a salient part of one's health plan are meant to be *observed*, not to rule your life. Growth and development are integral parts of human life — they give it meaning and purpose. Becoming regimented by rules and regulations eventually defeats the very purpose of the health plan. It's inadvisable to stick to any regimen one hundred per cent of the time. Life is a variable phenomenon.

Merely being in the finest physical condition is no assurance that you are healthy. You have needs and wants, and cling to aspirations and hopes for yourself and those you love. But an ability to meet these needs and wants, sometimes through planning but more often in adverse and unexpected situations, is an equally important part of your health. If you follow too rigid a lifestyle, your potential to meet adverse and unexpected conditions will be greatly hampered.

BECOMING HEALTHY

Western society is organized in such a way that we come to depend entirely on the medical establishment — doctors, pharmaceutical companies, hospitals and clinics — for solutions to our health problems. In fact, many people depend on these organizations to determine their health for them. But health is clearly a joint responsibility. There are some things which only a doctor can do, for he or she has trained for many years and there is no substitute for the skill and knowledge thus gained. On the other hand, there are things that only you can do for yourself, even if it is only implementing your doctor's advice. Becoming healthy and keeping well involve not only adopting living habits that prevent the onset of illness, but also knowing when to go to a doctor and how to use his or her services. By being aware of illnesses and diseases and by keeping informed we are more motivated to take care of ourselves when we feel fine. One of the regrettable characteristics of our normal attitude is that we do not want to be aware of illness and disease when we are not sick. We avoid thinking about it as much as we can and assume that we cannot become as seriously sick as someone else. As a result, when we are afflicted with a serious illness it hits us at many levels and we are emotionally devastated.

When we are not sick, there are many common health practices that lead to better health. Tibetan medical literature suggests the following guidelines:

Your Body Type and Functions

Know your body — its structure and functions. Study your body type and its digestion, circulation, stress levels and defense mechanisms.

The Environment and Where You Live

Be aware of conditions in the area where you live, such as the altitude, temperature, barometric pressure and humidity. Record these measurements for each season, and, more importantly, see how your body and its specific functions react to changes in these measurements. It may help to keep a diary.

Seasonal Influences

Study how each of the seasons affects your body and emotions. Does a cold wet winter, or a dry winter, produce depression, joint aches, poor digestion, etc.? Does a hot dry summer cause skin irritation, discomfort, etc.?

Your Constitutional Type

Take the constitutional typology test to determine your type. Use the results as a guideline in planning your diet and behavior.

Your Age

Age is an aspect of constitutional development. From the fetal period to age eight there is a very physical stage when the constitutional type called Water (Bagan) is most prominent in your development. Between eight and forty-five there is an extroverted stage wherein the Fire (Tripa) constitutional type dominates your development. Finally, beyond the age of forty-five there is an introverted stage wherein the Air (Lung) type is prominent in your development.

Constitutional Vulnerability or Weak Organs and Emotions

Find out which part of your body is generally the weakest and most vulnerable to illness or injury. For instance, you might find that your kidneys and urinary tract seem to be the most vulnerable organs of your body. Similarly, you might find that emotionally you tend to give up easily and despair.

This indicates that not only should you take extra precautions with regard to these organs but also with regard to related systems such as the spleen or the lymphatic and mucus systems.

Rates of Digestion and Absorption

By observing your digestive and eliminative functions you can be more selective in your diet. You will make more intelligent choices in your cooking and eating.

Body Weight and Strength

Find out what body weight and level of strength is appropriate for your height and age.

Nutrition

Over a two-week period, record the types of food that agree or do not agree with you. For instance, food types that cause an upset stomach, gas or bloating, or diarrhea are disagreeable and therefore inappropriate for your diet. Foods can be rendered good for you by proper preparation, the use of proper herbs and spices, etc.

Behavior

Consider how you think, emote, act and communicate, and then evaluate this behavior during your daily life. Include the way the seasons and the environment affect this behavior.

These areas are the basis for the constitutional typology test in Chapter 3, which will help determine the appropriate health plan for you. But in order to better understand the nature of the test and its results, let us first examine some of the fundamental principles of Tibetan medicine.

2
FUNDAMENTAL PRINCIPLES
OF TIBETAN MEDICINE

The Tibetan medical system is enormously rich and complex, but its fundamental principles can be quickly understood. In this chapter, principles such as the Five Elements, the Three Nepas, the Twenty Attributes and the Seven Tissues will be briefly introduced. The interrelatedness of these concepts will then be demonstrated.

THE FIVE ELEMENTS

The body is a fascinating and complex composition of what the Eastern medical systems call the Five Elements. From the body's major organs and systems such as the muscles, the skeleton, and the heart, to its smallest cellular structures, the Five Elements combine and interact to keep the body functioning well. In fact, the Buddhist and Vedic literatures on cosmology include elaborate descriptions of the natures and functions of the Five Elements, both in the environment and in the body.

Earth, Water, Fire, Air and Space — the Five Elements each have a distinct function in the body. The Earth element provides stability and structure, while the Water element provides moisture and smoothness. Growth, development, and the assimilation and absorption of food are all made possible by the Fire element. We are able to move our joints and muscles and to circulate blood and fluids because of the Air element. The Space element allows the other four elements the opportunity to interact and coexist.

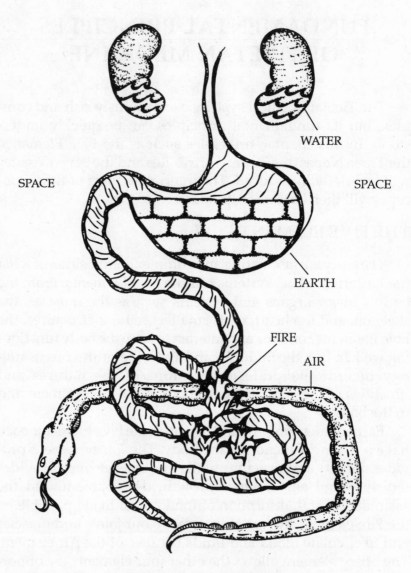

WATER

SPACE

SPACE

EARTH

FIRE

AIR

THE FIVE ELEMENTS

THE TWENTY ATTRIBUTES

In the Tibetan system there are ten pairs of attributes that can be used to characterize all animate and inanimate phenomena.

cold — hot
wet — dry
heavy — light
gross — subtle
dense — flowing
static — mobil
dull — sharp
soft — hard
smooth — rough
clear — cloudy

THE THREE NEPAS

The Tibetan medical system is based upon an understanding of the Nepas, the three principles which control the interactions and functions of the Five Elements. The Three Nepas can be considered both as energies and as physiological processes. They completely govern the body's physiology, psychology, and physiopathology. When they are in balance, health is assured; but when they are disturbed, disease and disorder will arise.

The Tibetan words for the Three Nepas are Lung (Air), Tripa (Fire), and Bagan (Water). These correspond to the Ayurvedic constitutional types of Vata (Air), Pitta (Fire) and Kapha (water).

Air (Lung)

Air (Lung, pronounced "loong"), is the energetic principle and physiological process concerned primarily with the workings of the nervous system, but it is also associated with the heart, the ears, the colon, the joints, and the texture of the skin.

Fire (Tripa)

Fire (Tripa, pronounced "treepa") is associated with the eyes, the liver, the gall bladder, the small intestine, and also with the workings of the vascular, endocrine, and secretory systems.

Water (Bagan)

Water (Bagan, pronounced "baygen") is associated with digestive and lymphatic systems, and in particular with the stomach, spleen, pancreas, urinary bladder and kidneys.

❀ ❀ ❀

To fully understand the Three Nepas, both their functions and their characteristics must be learned. First we will introduce these functions, then the twenty attributes by which the characteristics are described.

FUNCTIONS OF THE THREE NEPAS

Air (Lung)

Air (Lung) is concerned with movement, breathing, and all the senses. It ensures the balance of the other two Nepas, so an Air disorder is usually considered very severe.

Fire (Tripa)

Fire (Tripa) is concerned with digestion and the creation and maintenance of body heat. It also controls the assimilation and transformation of nutrients.

Water (Bagan)

Water (Bagan) is concerned with the structure and stability of the body, holding everything together and providing weight. It also ensures proper moisture, lubricating the body and protecting it from excess heat and irritation. Therefore, Water cools the heat of Fire and slows down the mobility of Air.

CHARACTERISTICS OF THE THREE NEPAS

Air (Lung)

Air (Lung) has six characteristics: **dry, light, cool, mobile, subtle,** and **hard.** When the body becomes imbalanced as a result of stress and tension, incorrect diet or other causes, Air may increase and, if not corrected, directly detectable symptoms having these six characteristics may arise. Symptoms with a **dry** character may include irritated skin, a dry mouth or tongue, or a foul temperament, while those with a **light** character can include forgetfulness, light-headedness or insomnia. Symptoms that are **mobile** include trembling, delirium, hysteria, and diffused pain and dizziness, and those that have a **subtle** character are blurred vision, ringing in the ears, and a pins-and-needles feeling. A **cool** symptom is the chills, and symptoms with a **hard** character include stiff joints and constipation.

Fire (Tripa) is **oily, sharp, malodorous, purging, hot, flowing** and **light.** When Fire is increased, its seven characteristics produce corresponding systems. **Hot** may produce symptoms of overheating and thirst, **sharp** may produce localized pain, the **light** characteristic may cause forgetfulness, and the **malodorous** may produce a rank-smelling stool or body odor. **Purging** and **flowing** may produce diarrhea or excessive mucus, and **oily** can produce an oily complexion.

Water (Bagan) is **cold, heavy, blunt, smooth, oily, stable** and **sticky.** When Water increases and becomes pathological, its seven characteristics may manifest as any of these kinds of symptoms. **Cold** symptoms are low body temperature, indigestion and a craving for a heat-producing diet. Symptoms with a **heavy** character are lethargy, mental dullness, sleepiness and slow recovery time, while those with a **smooth** character consist in having a smooth, cool tongue and dull pains. **Blunt** symptoms are slowly developing, while a **stable** symptom is localized and unchanging. **Sticky** symptoms may include cohesive urine, sweat and sputum.

Air and Water have **cold** in common; however, there is a difference. Air is actually more on the tepid side, and here **cold** simply means not **hot,** as found in Fire. Similarly, though Fire and Water both have the **oily** characteristic in common, they are not quite the same. Fire has a lighter, drier, less greasy and more penetrating type of the **oily** characteristic than is found in Water. Both Air and Fire have the **light** characteristic in common. Again, however, these are not quite the same. The **light** in Air is more diffused and volatile, while in Fire it is localized and penetrating.

THE TWENTY FUNDAMENTAL ATTRIBUTES AND HOW THEY AFFECT THE THREE NEPAS

① Primary Effect   ② Secondary Effect   ③ Minimal Effect

Attribute	Air (Lung)	Fire (Tripa)	Water (Bagan)
Hot	② decreases	③ increases	① decreases
Cold	② increases	③ decreases	① increases
Wet	① decreases	② decreases	③ increases
Dry	① increases	② increases	③ decreases
Heavy	① decreases	② decreases	③ increases
Light	① increases	② increases	③ decreases
Mass	① decreases	② decreases	③ increases
Subtle	① increases	② increases	③ decreases
Dense	① decreases	② decreases	③ increases
Flowing	① decreases	③ increases	② decreases
Mobile	① increases	② increases	③ decreases
Static	① decreases	② decreases	③ increases
Dullness	① decreases	② decreases	③ increases
Sharp	② increases	① increases	③ decreases
Smooth	③ decreases	② increases	① increases
Rough	③ increases	② decreases	① decreases
Clear	① increases	② increases	③ decreases
Cloudy	① decreases	② decreases	③ increases
Soft	③ decreases	② increases	① increases
Hard	① increases	③ decreases	② decreases

SITES OF THE THREE NEPAS

Each of the Three Nepas is associated with certain areas of the body, and it is in these areas that a Nepa disorder of a particular kind is likely to manifest. These locations should be taken into account when characterizing signs and symptoms.

Air (Lung)

Air (Lung) is associated with the colon, thighs, hips, ears, joints, bones and skin. The locations of Fire (Tripa) are the small intestine, gall bladder, liver, sweat glands, blood, eyes and stomach. Water (Bagan) is associated with the stomach, spleen, kidneys, pancreas, urinary bladder, adipose tissues, chest, head, throat, nose, tongue and lymph glands.

SIGNS AND SYMPTOMS OF THE THREE NEPAS

There are many signs and symptoms of poor health, and they can all be associated with one or more of the twenty attributes. However, in practice it is much more beneficial to relate a group of these signs and symptoms to one of the Three Nepas. Of course, most of these signs and symptoms will have the characteristics found in the particular Nepa. In other words, an Air (Lung) disorder will have signs and symptoms that are **dry, light, cool, mobile, subtle** or **hard.**

Air (Lung)

Signs and symptoms of Air (Lung) disorder are: frequent sighing, mental wandering and distraction, dizziness, ringing in the ears, diffused pain, muscular tension, poor circulation, cold extremities, tremors, chills, stiffness and difficulty in movement, lethargy, pain in the joints, frequent pins and needles sensation, starry eyes, goose pimples, insomnia or disturbed sleep and dreams, pains in either the lower skull, chest or jaws, dry heaves, gas or a rumbling sound in the abdomen, and constipation.

Fire (Tripa)

Signs and symptoms of Fire (Tripa) disorder are: diarrhea, vomiting, itchy skin, intense thirst, bitter taste in the mouth, fever, sleeplessness, strong odor of the urine and stool, headaches, nausea, and discomfort in the liver and gall bladder regions.

Water (Bagan)

Signs and symptoms of Water (Bagan) disorder are: pale complexion and gums, excess mucus, lethargy, poor appetite, low body temperature, indigestion, slow digestion, discomfort in the lower back or kidney region, fluid retention and puffiness, sleepiness, and poor memory and dullness.

AGGRAVATING FACTORS
FOR THE THREE NEPAS

FACTORS THAT PROMOTE AIR (LUNG) IMBALANCE		
DIET		
Tastes:	Bitter	Pungent	Astringent
Attributes:	Light	Dry	Rough
Foods:	Raw or Yellow Vegetables		
	Light Millet		
	Caffeine		
	Light Cereals		
	Pork		
	Refined Sugar		
BEHAVIOR		
Attributes:	Light	Mobile	Rough
Activities:	Irregular Sleeping or Eating Patterns		
	Excessive Mental, Verbal, or Physical Exertion		
	Stress and Strain		
Season:	Early Summer		

FACTORS THAT PROMOTE FIRE (TRIPA) IMBALANCE

DIET

Tastes:	Sour	Pungent	Salty	
Attributes:	Hot	Sharp	Oily	Light
Foods:	Animal Proteins			
	Fried or Fatty Foods			
	Eggs			
	Mutton			
	Spicy Foods			
	Salt			
	Beef			
	Alcohol			

BEHAVIOR

Attributes:	Hot	Oily
Activites:	Strenuous Physical Labor or Strain on the Liver	
	New Environments or Threatening Situations	
Season:	Late Summer	

FACTORS THAT PROMOTE WATER (BAGAN) IMBALANCE

DIET

Tastes:	Sweet	Salty	
Attributes:	Heavy	Cold	Wet
Foods:	Raw, Cold or Heavy Cireals and Vegetables		
	Dairy Products		

BEHAVIOR

Attributes:	Heavy	Static
Activities:	Lack or Physical Exercise	
	Lack of Mental, Verbal, or Physical Stimulation	
	Depressing Activities	
Season:	Winter and Spring	

THE SEVEN TISSUES

There are seven principal pathways through which the body receives nourishment. When they are free from blockages and subtle energy losses, growth and health can be maintained; otherwise, disease may occur. The Seven Tissues are plasma, blood, muscle, adipose tissue, bone, marrow and seminal fluid. Each of these must exist in just the right proportions in the body. For instance, if there is excess adipose tissue, obesity, fatigue, sexual debility or lethargy may arise. However, if there is not enough adipose tissue the nails and teeth may become brittle, joints may crack, and emaciation may occur.

THE THREE BODY WASTES

The body expels waste in three forms: urine, feces and sweat. Heat as well as toxic substances are eliminated in these forms, and it is imperative that the pathways of their release be free and flowing. Bowel movements and urination should be regular and sweating should happen during regular exercise.

THE DIGESTIVE FIRE

When the digestive fire is sufficient, the body will function well by producing just the right amount of heat to carry out digestion without destroying the nutrients. In addition, this heat destroys toxins that might otherwise build up. The digestive fire has all the characteristics of the fire element: it is **hot, dry, light, mobile, subtle** and **sharp.** There are four degrees of digestive fire: high, low, variable and balanced. Balanced is of course the most desirable.

Fire (Tripa)

People of the type generally have a high digestive fire; their digestion is strong and their appetites are good.

Water (Bagan)

Water (Bagan) types have a low degree of digestive fire which causes a slow metabolism and a tendency to gain weight.

Air (Lung)

In the case of Air (Lung) types, the digestive fire is variable, depending on their diet, behavior and mood. As a result, sometimes their digestion is active while sometimes it is quite poor.

3
THE TIBETAN CONSTITUTIONAL
TYPOLOGY TEST

FOUR BASIC STEPS
TOWARD YOUR HEALTH PLAN

The first step toward your health plan is to know as much as you can about yourself. You need to review your medical history carefully — recent or present health conditions and then your constitutional typology. The Tibetan constitutional typology test is an effective evaluation technique for determining your type.

The second step is to learn what kind of behavior (including mental, physical and communicative) is appropriate and healthy in terms of your constitutional typology. By studying the behavioral recommendations outlined in this book, you can start to formulate a health plan. The health plan needs to be constantly updated and nourished as one grows, changes and matures.

The third step requires that you explore what type of nutrition is most healthy for you. Chapter 5 outlines what types of foods are healthy, how much you should eat, and how to prepare and combine herbs and spices to form a balanced diet.

The fourth step is to be realistic in your planning. There are general or commonly shared health goals and there are specific or individual health goals. A common goal to which all of us aspire is the enjoyment of prolonged good health. An increased life span and general good health are probably the most common and basic goals. Individual health goals, on the other hand, are specific to each individual. In addition to the common goals of good health and long life, you will need to think about personal health issues such as (for example) excess

body weight, a hyperthyroid condition, poor metabolic profile, or a hormonal dysfunction. These health conditions will
become the basis for your personal health goals. You need to
work out a strategy in addition to the guidelines given here in
this book for your general health plan, taking into account
your individual health conditions as part of that plan.

For many of us, the above health goals have meaning only
when we include psychological and spiritual goals. What is
the purpose of a healthy and robust body? Is it just to look after
our physical and psychological needs and to feel good about
ourselves, or do we have other responsibilities and dimen-
sions as unique individuals?

CONSTITUTIONAL TYPOLOGIES

The constitutional typology test consists of two major
parts: one to determine your body type and another to determine your psychological profile. The constitutional typology
test is fairly simple and aimed at giving a general picture of
you as a person. Apart from its benefits in helping to plan your
health program, the constitutional typology test can assist
immensely in determining the line of treatment in case of a
disorder. For instance, if a Air (Lung) person and a Fire (Tripa)
person both suffer from non-specific symptom patterns such
as headaches, constipation, dizziness and so forth, the Tibetan
physician will treat the Air (Lung) client as suffering from a
more severe condition than the Fire (Tripa) client, even though
both have the same signs and symptoms. This is because the
Air (Lung) type is inherently more anxious and tense than the
Fire (Tripa) type, and therefore these stress symptoms have a
deeper structural meaning and more potential to create full-
blown psychological disorders than they would for the Fire
(Tripa) type. In Tibet, many patients would know their constitutional type and, upon visiting a physician, the first thing they
would do would be to tell him their type.

To assess your body type, it is important to first determine
what the average body type profile is like in your society. There
are seven body types, which are often subsumed into just the
first three. The three major typologies are Air (Lung), Fire

(Tripa), and Water (Bagan), which correspond to ectomorph, mesomorph, and endomorph respectively. The remaining four types are combinations of these three.

Air (Lung) or Ectomorph Type

BODY:	Tall, lean physique with a short trunk, long extremities, and a long, thin neck
FACE:	Small, elongated skull; narrow forehead, sharp nose and projecting ears; mostly blue eyes; light-colored, thin and soft hair
CHEST:	Narrow and drooping shoulders; narrow, depressed chest with prominent scapulae
ABDOMEN:	Small, flat and hard
EXTREMITIES:	Long and thin
GENITALS:	Long, thin penis and elongated scrotum; poorly developed vagina, small breasts; irregular and prolonged menstrual problems
MUSCLES:	Generally weak, with poor circulation
SKIN:	Dry, rough, and discolored
BODY FUNCTIONS:	Muscular, nervous, and sensory responses to stimulation are rapid but short-lived; the body is prone to rapid exhaustion and low resistance. The predominant physiological function is that of the nervous system; the digestive tract is very sensitive to external influences; sex drive fluctuates and is normally weak

Fire (Tripa) or Mesomorph Type

BODY:	Strong and muscular, with good general tone; well proportioned and of medium height
FACE:	Short skull with wide forehead, protruding eyebrows, round nose, dark eyes and thick, coarse hair
CHEST:	Well developed and proportioned
ABDOMEN:	Small and muscular
EXTREMITIES:	Well proportioned and strong
GENITALS:	Thick and developed penis, contracted and hard scrotum; female organs are strong and of medium size
MUSCLES:	Compact and strong, with good circulation

SKIN:	Elastic, thick and of olive complexion
BODY FUNCTIONS:	Muscular, nervous and sensory responses to stimulation are rapid and lasting; resistance is good. The chief physiological activities are those of the endocrine and secretory organs. In women, menstruation, pregnancy and delivery are usually normal. This type has the best physique

Water (Bagan) or Endomorph Type

BODY:	Weak muscles, strong bones of medium tone; heavy, short physique tending to retain fluid and fat
FACE:	Large, elongated head with narrow forehead, small eyes, thick eyelids, wide nose and thick lips, short and heavy neck, and soft, thick hair
CHEST:	Round and soft shoulders
ABDOMEN:	Large and soft
EXTREMITIES:	Thick and short
GENITALS:	Thick and short penis, heavy and thick scrotum; female organs are well developed; tendency to heavy menstruation
MUSCLES:	Soft and flabby, with poor circulation
SKIN:	Pale and soft
BODY FUNCTIONS:	Muscular, nervous and sensory responses to stimulation are slow and lethargic; resistance is moderate. The chief physiological activities are those of the lymphatic system and digestive tract

It is unlikely that any individual will have *all* the individual features of any one of the three body types. To determine your body type, see whether your major features of face, height and weight match one of the three types. In this evaluation, an average person of Fire (Tripa) type in your community should be used as a basis for determining your own body type. This way, a more accurate assessment is possible.

PSYCHOLOGICAL PROFILES

The second part of the test involves a description of the personality traits for each of the three types.

Air (Lung) Psychological Profile

MOOD: Depressive, anxious; moods change from one extreme to another — from depression to euphoria, love to hate, mercy to contempt

WILL: Idealistic but rarely carries a task to completion, often because of a lack of self-esteem and confidence. Emotionally unstable and easily affected by situations and circumstances

EGO: Egotism is often the main feature of the psychological make-up, owing to a sense of threat from others (typically Tripa personalities) whom he or she may envy and consider stronger and more mature

INTELLIGENCE: Highly intelligent and quick to learn, but impractical.

EMOTION: Desirous and grasping, often resulting in frustration or fear of rejection and loss. Pleasure and pain are the chief sensation preoccupations

DEVIATIONS: Fear and complexes about sex and the opposite sex, often resulting in spiritual or sexual deviations. Women usually lack maternal feeling; pregnancy and childbirth are often not desired.

Fire (Tripa) Psychological Profile

MOOD: Aggressive, excitable, impulsive, materialistic, practical, calculating and often dictatorial

WILL: Strong will-power; optimistic; preoccupied with controlling situations and with organization; constantly changing to keep up with situations that are seen as threats.

EGO: Strong sense of the self as a permanent structure which is fortified by power, sex and wealth. Possesses an air of confidence and solidity visible even during casual conversation. Avoids spiritual issues or dismisses them as silly or immaterial; instantly turns away from conversations that remind him or her of the impermanence of the world.

INTELLIGENCE: Scheming and compulsive; thinks in terms of ends and means, sequences and the order of carrying out a function. Constantly searching for a model, a point of reference to measure against as well as to reassure himself or herself that he or she is doing well.

EMOTION: Envy and jealousy are deep-rooted, and behavior revolves around these emotions. A poor loser, he or she can manifest aggressive behavior when his or her world view is threatened. Preoccupation with one's own importance is often seen in dedication to appearance and body. Probably the healthiest type, with an enormous amount of energy which, unfortunately, is often spent wastefully. While physically healthy, the immune system may be poor because he or she is constantly taxing his or her body and expending energy; even minor infections can become threatening.

DEVIATIONS: Sadistic, raging narcissism, self-cherising, self-centered behavior

Water (Bagan) Psychological Profile

MOOD: Warm-hearted, stable, easy-going, lively, carefree and pleasure-loving.

WILL: Weak and leisure-oriented; slow to grasp ideas; resistant to change and putting ideas into action; procrastinates.

EGO: No dominant features; concept of self revolves around comfort and peaceful surroundings.

INTELLIGENCE: Average; lacks great aspirations.

EMOTION: Resistant to any major change in life situation; rigid adherence to the status quo; a dull neutrality; unresponsive to new ideas and stimulations; preoccupied with nutrition; shows the closest behavioral patterns to those of a "primitive" type. Though striking in appearance, warm and straightforward and without hypocrisy, good-natured and understanding, he or she has fixed ideas and is self-righteous. Dirty dishes pile up, work is left incomplete, and close personal relationships are neglected.

DEVIATIONS: Fun and pleasure; over-indulgence in food; most minimal sexual deviations.

THE TIBETAN CONSTITUTIONAL TYPOLOGY TEST

The first seven sections of this test focus on physical characteristics and environmental influences. The remaining sections focus primarily on the psychological and spiritual components of the individual. Many of the questions in these sections deal with the darker aspects of human nature, to get a better assessment of the personality. These questions are not meant to imply that these personality aspects are negative shortcomings from which you, personally, suffer.

Instructions

Answer the questions in each section by drawing a circle around the letter preceding the answer you choose. The test should not be taken when you are under stress or when you are suffering from any kind of illness.

SECTION I.
W — *Are you between five and twenty years old?*
    a. Yes
    b. No

F — *Are you between twenty-five and sixty years old?*
    a. Yes
    b. No

A — *Are you over sixty years old?*
    a. Yes
    b. No

SECTION II.
Which body type fits you most closely?
A — Air (Lung) or Ectomorph
F — Fire (Tripa) or Mesomorph
W — Water (Bagan) or Endomorph

SECTION III.
Which of the following environments or climates agrees with your health?
A — A hot and moderately dry climate
F — A cold and wet climate
W — A cool and dry climate

Which of the following climates generally does not agree with your health?
A — A cool and dry climate
F — A hot and dry climate
W — A cold and wet climate

SECTION IV.
Which of the following seasons agrees with your health?
A — Autumn
F — Winter and Spring
W — Summer

Which of the following does not agree with your health?
A — Summer
F — Autumn
W — Winter and Spring

SECTION V.
During which part of a normal day (for you) do you feel best with respect to your body and health?
A — Afternoon between noon and 3:00 and night between midnight and 2:00 A.M.
F — Morning from 8:00 to 11:00 and night between 8:00 and midnight
W — Early morning before 7:00 A.M. and evening between 5:00 and 8:00 P.M.
(These hours may vary among individuals, so give or take an hour from those listed.)

During which part of a normal day (for you) do you not feel up to the mark?

A — Early morning before 7:00 A.M. and evening between 5:00 and 8:00 P.M.

F — Afternoon between noon and 3:00 and night between midnight and 2:00 A.M.

W — Morning from 8:00 to 11:00 and night between 8:00 and midnight

SECTION VI.

When do you generally feel better?

A — Immediately after eating

F — Two to four hours after eating your normal meal

W — On an empty stomach and after eating very small, light meals

When do you generally feel worse?

A — On an empty stomach

F — Two to four hours after eating your normal meal

W — Immediately after eating

SECTION VII.

Constitutionally, which part of your body feels weakest and most prone to ailments?

A — Lower part of body (entire body below the navel, including legs and feet)

F — Middle part of body (entire body between heart and navel)

W — Upper part of body (entire body above the heart, including head)

Constitutionally, which part of your body feels healthiest and most free from ailments?

A — Middle part of body

F — Upper part of body

W — Lower part of body

How much exercise do your prefer?
A — Light exercise, not done regularly
F — Competitive and strenuous exercise, done regularly
    and with zeal
W — None or very little

What is your sleeping pattern like?
A — Disturbed sleep pattern
F — Need little sleep
W — Heavy and prolonged

When under stress and tension, which of the following symptoms do you tend to experience?

A	F	W
muscular tension	localized pain	dullness & heaviness
tension headache	migraine	sleepiness
ringing in ears	nausea	cold hands & feet
hyperventilation	heat in body	sluggishness
gas	acidity	fullness in stomach
constipation	diarrhea	poor digestion

(It is likely that you experience symptoms from all three categories; however, choose only the set of symptoms that seems to be most noticeable and consistent.)

SECTION VIII.

Which of the following psychological symptoms do you generally experience when under stress and tension?

A	F	W
nervousness/anxiety	anger	resistance
restlessness	aggression	denial
constant worry/brooding	irritability	procrastination
thinking too much	harsh and abusive	withdrawn
grieving	violent	silent and sullen
easily upset	high-strung	closed-minded
mood swings	jealous	confused, forgetful

(Since it is likely that you experience symptoms from all three categories, try to choose the category with the most significant symptoms for you.)

SECTION IX.
Emotional symptoms you generally experience:

A	F	W
excitement	aggression	stable and sedating
greed	vengeance	concealment
pretension	envy	indifference

(Answer this question in the same manner as you answered those in Section VIII.)

SECTION X.
Which of the following belief systems do you generally follow?
A — Abstract, emotional and intense belief system
F — Concrete, materially oriented belief system
W — Generic or none

SECTION XI.
How are your concentration skills?
A — Easily distracted and cannot concentrate on an object for a long time (except sexual objects)
F — Focused; good concentration, primarily on materially oriented objects and goals
W — Poor concentration due to dullness and indifference

SECTION XII.
What is your spiritual practice like?
A — Very important to you
F — Not absolutely essential
W — You recognize its importance but don't really practice

Determining Your Type

Add up all the circled letters. The highest number of answers for any one letter indicates your primary constitutional typology. The second highest indicates your secondary typology.

For example, if you score 20 A's and 16 F's, then your constitutional typology is Air–Fire (Lung-Tripa).

4
DIAGNOSIS

INTRODUCTION

When we talk about diagnosis in the West, we assume that the person already has a manifest complaint or disorder. The physician's job, then, is to match the signs and symptoms that the client complains about with those that he finds, and associate them with a particular disorder. In Tibetan medicine, however, we think about diagnosis in terms of measuring the balance between the vital body organs and the systems that govern them. By using the three-humor and the hot-cold model, the Tibetan physician analyzes what is wrong with the client by closely monitoring the interaction between the various organs and functions of the body.

To determine what the condition of the body is in general, you must observe the minutest details about the client's body, beginning with the eyes, tongue, ears, nose and skin, then feeling the abdomen, pressing acupressure points, and examining excretory discharges from the body such as sputum, feces and urine. After you have a very clear picture of the client's general condition, you begin to question him or her about the complaint. The signs that you discover by using a diagnostic procedure as well as the symptoms that the client complains about are carefully evaluated in light of your knowledge of symptomatology and specific disorders. This part of evaluation — observing signs and symptoms and fitting them correctly into the disorder classification — is crucial, particularly for differential diagnosis. Without training in symptomatology and disorders, the physician cannot make instant and correct diagnoses when called upon in a clinical situation.

The next step is to organize the clinical information you have gathered, to ensure that it is consistent with your line of assessment. For instance, if the pulse indicates an inflammatory condition, the characteristics of the urine, eyes, and tongue, as well as the answers to your questioning, must also indicate inflammation. When they do not correspond, such as when the urine shows inflammation but the pulse does not, both should be re-examined to analyze for the presence of transient, superficial imbalances or other complications. There may be several pathological as well as constitutional factors that could be responsible for the inconsistency, and it is the job of the physician to work out what is involved. The finding of a transient cold imbalance such as indigestion, for instance, can be responsible for the difference in the clinical features of urine and pulse.

Ultimately the ability of the physician to question the client efficiently, organize the information, and interpret the signs and symptoms that the client complains about is the most crucial diagnostic procedure. Otherwise, by merely reading the pulse, studying the urine, and examining the body, you will miss part of the total picture and often end up with an incomplete or even incorrect diagnosis. The diagnostic procedures, in addition to their use in determining an imbalance or pathological condition, can also be used to measure your state of health at any given time. A day-to-day observation of the pulse, urine, tongue, face, eyes, lips and skin gives an indication of the present condition of the body. By regularly making these observations, pathological symptoms and imbalances can be detected early and preventative measures taken.

To be an effective diagnostician, however, you must be sensitive and perceptive. Not only must you have sharp eyes, nose, and sensitive fingers with which to feel, but you must be perceptive in assessing people by means of their expressions and gestures, how they sit and dress, and how they relate to you and others. This kind of skill does not come easily to everyone, nor can it be entirely learned, for a person needs to be truly involved with what he is doing and truly care about and empathize with the situations of his or her clients. Only then will the client open up and express himself or herself in new ways, providing insights into his or her condition and emotions.

Such skills are crucial for a Tibetan physician because he or she is responsible in the final analysis for treatment of the client. He or she does not have sophisticated support systems such as high-tech laboratories or trained staff to carry out expensive and complex diagnostic tests and procedures. A Tibetan physician has to depend upon himself or herself, along with his or her training and empathy for the client.

TIBETAN DIAGNOSTIC PROCEDURE

How is a client diagnosed and what are the procedures the Tibetan physician follows when a client comes into the clinic? Following is an outline of the diagnostic procedures and stages:

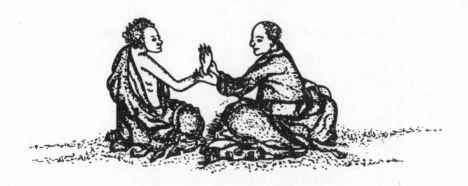

1. EXAMINATION OF THE RADIAL ARTERY PULSE ON BOTH OF THE CLIENT'S WRISTS

2. EXAMINATION OF THE CLIENT'S URINE IN CLEAR, BRIGHT LIGHT

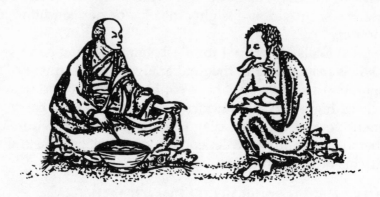

3. PHYSICAL EXAMINATION
- Examination of the five sensory organs
  1. Tongue
  2. Eyes
  3. Ears
  4. Nose and lips
  5. Skin

- Functional relationship between the five sense and their objects
  1. Taste
  2. Shapes and colors
  3. Sounds
  4. Odors
  5. Sensations

- Examination of the five excretory matters
  1. Sputum
  2. Vomit
  3. Urine
  4. Blood composition
  5. Feces

- Examination of the abdomen and acupressure points
  1. Palpating the abdomen
  2. Feeling acupressure points

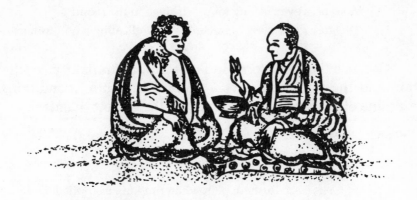

4. QUESTIONING AND HISTORY
- Questions about diet
- Questions about behavior and psychological and emotional structures
- Questions about reaction to medication

HOW TO TAKE THE PULSE

Using his senses as an extension of his intelligence, the Tibetan physician learns how to fathom the inner world of his clients. Using his eyes, ears, and nose, he studies and assesses the meaning of superficial manifestations of internal body events. When feeling for pulses, he taps even more deeply into the human body and is in touch with the circulation of energy and blood that has contacted all parts of the body. By applying varying degrees of pressure and feeling the radial artery of a client at specific positions, he is able to monitor the functions of the body in general as well as have access to the activities of specific systems and organs. The pulse can tell you much about the client and his or her condition, but it is not always accurate by itself. One must learn to distinguish the true from the false by learning to organize and interpret findings from other modalities such as the tongue, eyes, urine, sputum, skin, etc., in order to arrive at the right answer. For instance, a client comes to you with the following:

Symptoms: Fever, aching joints, dryness in the mouth
Signs: Pulse slow, weak and thin, indicating a non-inflammatory cold condition

Because the symptoms indicate an inflammatory condition and the pulse indicates a non-inflammatory condition,
examine other modalities to arrive at the correct diagnosis.

PHYSICAL SYMPTOMS:
Urine: Turbid, dark and odorous
Tongue: Red and dry
EYES: Face flushed; pain when pressure is applied

QUESTIONING:
Diet: Heat-producing foods such as spices, meat, wine,
and greasy, oily foods cause discomfort and aggravate the condition. Cold-producing foods such as
salads, the nightshade family, grains, cereals, water
and curd produce relief.
Seasonal In early summer, autumn, and afternoons, the con-
Reactions: dition is aggravated. In winter, spring, mornings
and evenings, the condition improves.
Behavior: Strenuous activities, anger, and aggressive behavior aggravate the condition. Relaxation, rest, and
soothing or cooling activities relieve the condition.

Final diagnosis, based on the above signs and symptoms:
Primary hot or cold inflammatory disorder with possible
secondary cold condition.

What the pulse tells us:
1. It gives us a standard of health
2. It detects any deviation from that standard.

How does it do this?
1. It defines the location of important parts of the body
(upper, middle and lower)
2. It defines the physiology of the body at any one point
(blood, energy and organs)

3. It defines the following functions: circulation, respiration, digestion and the nervous system
4. It defines individual characteristics of normality:

Pulse rate: Depends on age
  Volume: Depends on constitutional predisposition
  Depths: Superficial and deep
  Strength: Depends on physical build
Relationship: The parts of the pulse under each fingertip
     should be balanced and even

Conditions for Taking the Pulse

The pulse can reveal both pathological and constitutional information about the client. In order to obtain information about the person's constitution, the person must be basically in a healthy state, since any major pathological condition from which he may be suffering will make it exceedingly difficult for the physician to read his constitutional pulse accurately. Make sure that the client is relaxed and breathing normally. To avoid strain and discomfort, make sure both of you are sitting on seats of equal height and place a cushion under the client's arm. Before the pulse is read, the client should routinely be questioned about any abnormal or extreme diet or behavior patterns during the past three days, since these factors may easily affect the pulse.

Method for Taking the Pulse

The pulse is taken at both radial arteries on the client's wrists in turn, with the right hand of the physician on the left wrist of the client and the left hand on the right wrist of the client. The pulse should be taken distal to proximal on each arm (see diagrams). There are two main positions the physician must use. First is the superficial, which means the minimal pressure of his three middle fingertips on the radial artery skin surface, just enough pressure to feel the pulse at the skin level. This position is held for ten or more seconds and it is important to do so since it may take some time to pick up the pulse beat at this level. If the pulse beat at this level is strong, bulky and variant in nature, then stay on it for some time in order to determine its actual character. This is again vital because sometimes the pulse may initially appear strong and bulky, but, as you stay on it, it may change to a tighter and more consistent beat.

The deep pulse is similar to the superficial pulse, except that you apply sufficient pressure to feel the pulse at the level of the bone and muscles in the wrist. Note that the deep pulse will be different because you are diagnosing deep internal organs rather than superficial organs such as the skin and muscles.

PHYSICIAN'S LEFT-HAND FINGERS:

	Upper	Lower
Index finger:	lungs	large intestine
Middle finger:	liver	gall bladder
Ring finger:	right kidney	urinary bladder

PHYSICIAN'S RIGHT-HAND FINGERS:

	Upper	Lower
Index finger:	heart	small intestine
Middle finger:	spleen	stomach
Ring finger:	left kidney	reproductive organs

TYPES OF PULSES
Healthy Pulse

A healthy pulse beats five times during one respiratory cycle (inhalation and exhalation), or about seventy-five times per minute, i.e. five to six beats in five seconds. The pulse should be uniform in rate, depth, volume, shape, strength, and tensity under all the physician's fingers. Any inconsistency in the pulse will indicate an imbalance or disorder of some kind. For instance, if the tensity of the pulse is hard and tight, an inflammatory or hot imbalance or disorder is present, even though other clinical features of the pulse — such as rate, depth, shape and strength — are uniform.

Since the pulse is easily affected by transitory factors such as breathing, stress, food and tension, the time spent on reading the pulse should be at least four or five minutes. This will allow the fingertips to recognize the superficial pulse beats and distinguish them from the real pulse, which can gradually be picked up.

Unhealthy Pulse

An unhealthy pulse is determined at three levels: the general or humoral (superficial), hot/cold (medium), and the specific organ (deep) levels.

THE SIX GENERAL HUMORAL PULSES OF IMBALANCE

These six pulses are read under all the fingertips and determine the deviation from the normal standard of health. While they indicate both imbalances and pathological states, the humoral pulses especially tell us about the general condition of the person and indicate any condition that may lead to a disorder. The person is then able to take preventative measures to avoid such a disorder. The six pulses are Wind (Air), Bile (Fire), Phlegm (Water), Wind-Bile (Air-Fire), Phlegm-Wind (Water-Air) and Phlegm-Bile (Water-Fire).

General Wind Pulse (Air)

At the superficial or skin level, the pulse is felt easily (sometimes strongly and sometimes a little weaker). However, when pressure is applied, it instantly comes to a complete stop and beats again only when the radial artery is released. Any resistance to the pressure indicates a contrary condition.

General Bile Pulse (Fire)

This type of pulse is thin and fast at the superficial level and gets tighter and more taut at the deep level. Generally the pulse rate is over seven beats in five seconds.

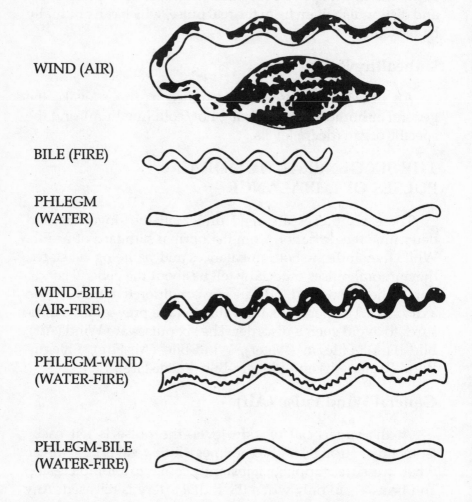

WIND (AIR)

BILE (FIRE)

PHLEGM
(WATER)

WIND-BILE
(AIR-FIRE)

PHLEGM-WIND
(WATER-FIRE)

PHLEGM-BILE
(WATER-FIRE)

PULSE CATEGORIES

General Phlegm Pulse (Water)

The phlegm pulse is barely even present at the superficial level; at the deep level, a slow, weak pulse is felt. The pulse rate is below five beats in five seconds.

Wind-Bile Pulse (Air-Fire)

The wind-bile pulse has characteristics of both the general wind and bile pulses. It is fast (more than six beats in five seconds) and slightly thin at the superficial level. When pressure is applied, it stops instantly. When pressure on the artery is released, the pulse beats at its original fast speed.

Phlegm-Bile Pulse (Water-Fire)

The phlegm-bile pulse is slow and weak at the superficial level, like the general phlegm pulse; however, at the deep level it is tight and hard and beats slightly faster.

Phlegm-Wind Pulse (Water-Air)

This type of pulse is slow and weak at the superficial level and stops when pressure is applied to the artery. The pulse rate is generally below six beats in five seconds.

❀ ❀ ❀

THE GENERAL HOT AND COLD IMBALANCE PULSES

This pulse is measured between the superficial and deep pulses. It describes the circulation of the blood. Following are the twelve major pulses of hot and cold imbalance:

Characteristic	Cold Imbalance	Hot Imbalance
Strength	Weak	Strong
Depth	Superficial	Deep
Volume	Declining	Pounding
Rate	Slow	Fast
Shape	Loose	Tight
Tensity	Empty	Hard & Tight

HOW TO ANALYZE URINE

The practice of healing is a very personal art and skill — an intense meeting of minds to solve a physical and emotional problem. The different forms of diagnosis in the Tibetan system are extremely useful tools in the diagnosis of a problem. As can be clearly seen from the section on pulse diagnosis, the basic skills can be learned fairly easily and with sufficient depth to be useful as a self-help technique for keeping tabs on our own health status. Urinalysis is used to confirm our findings from the pulse, to pick up factors missed in pulse diagnosis, and above all to determine the line of treatment. As with pulse diagnosis, I will present the basic steps of urinalysis for use in self-diagnosis. The basic skills can be acquired after a few months of practice and observation; however, the use of these techniques in clinical practice requires supervision and years of experience.

Conditions for Analyzing Urine

To take your pulse or analyze your urine, you need to comply with behavioral and dietary observances for at least two or three days before reading the pulse or urine. In short, these compliances mean that you should avoid any abnormal behavior or dietary abnormalities. Do not overeat or over-indulge in any activity during those two or three days. Above all, do not eat, drink or do anything which you normally don't. For instance, if you don't ordinarily eat meat, then certainly do not do so during these two or three days.

Since the urine changes its composition depending on your diet and behavior, any diet or behavior which is engaged in to excess will change the urine and prevent you from getting an accurate reading.

Observances Before Taking Urine

One should avoid the foods which aggravate one's constitutional typology:

Excessive Air (Lung) Foods (or Behavior):
- Light, mobile, dry and bitter tasting foods, such as light green raw vegetables
- Drinking strong tea
- Intense stress

Excessive Fire (Tripa) Foods:
- Heavy, wet, stagnating, sweet foods such as sugar and curd

Excessive Water (Bagan) Foods:
- Hot, oily, sharp, or hot and sour tasting foods
- Sour, acidic, fermented foods such as blue cheese, fatty foods, spicy and oily foods

The chief compliances to be observed are as follows:
- Avoid strong tea and light green vegetables
- Avoid excessively rich, oily foods
- Avoid excessive simple carbohydrates such as sugar
- Avoid excessive fluid intake
- Avoid sexual intercourse
- Avoid irregular sleeping patterns
- Avoid excessive stress

Clinical Features of Urine

The nine major features of urine which you must examine in order to use it as a clinical diagnostic tool are as follows:

- Color
- Odor
- Steam (when urine is fresh)
- Bubbles
- Cloudy, creamy, mucus-like formations (albumin)
- Formations of stringy sediment (chyle)
- The time when urine color and temperature change
- The clinical features of urine when it is cold

To use the urine for basic assessment purposes, the color, odor, bubbles, albumin, chyle, and the way it changes are sufficient.

Air (Lung) Urine

Color:	Bluish water, transparent
Odor:	Minimal or none
Bubbles:	Large, "the size of an ox's eye," appearing erratically on the surface of the urine
Cloudy formation:	None
Stringy formations:	Minimal, thin, or oily cream. None at all on the surface of the urine.
Sediments:	Minimal to moderate deposits, shaped like strands of hair
Rate of discoloration:	After urine cools, it dilutes and turns watery
Way change takes place:	Erratic and irregular
Characteristics of urine when cold:	Diluted and watery, with large bubbles that disappear slowly

Fire (Tripa) Urine

Color:	Yellow, orangeish, reddish and turbid
Odor:	Malodorous, pungent, foul
Bubbles:	Small bubbles that disappear instantly after stirring

Cloudy formation:	Thick, abundant
Stringy formations:	Thick, single units in the center and on the surface of the urine
Sediments:	Urine is murky, turbid and often has a cloudy deposit
Rate of discoloration:	Before urine turns cold
Way change takes place:	From the lower level towards the surface
Characteristics of urine when cold:	Turbid and reddish-yellow, with small bubbles that disappear instantly after stirring

Water (Bagan) Urine

Color:	White
Odor:	Minimal or none
Bubbles:	Small, congested, profuse, sticky, standing for a long time after stirring
Cloudy formation:	Minimal or none
Stringy formations:	Minimal or none
Sediments:	Minimal, or sometimes sand-like in kidney or metabolic disorders
Rate of discoloration:	Much after urine is cold
Way change takes place:	From the outside towards the center
Characteristics of urine when cold:	White, generally clear, congested, with increasing bubbles that persist or surface

The urine is best examined when it is fresh. If it is not fresh, then it should be examined when lukewarm or cold. Cold urine that has stood for eight to ten hours may also be examined in order to determine the client's constitutional and pathological conditions. The best time to examine the urine is before breakfast. When this is not possible, the client may be examined during any time of the day before evening. The important thing is that any examination must be conducted on an empty stomach.

Take the second half of your first morning urine before breakfast. Put it in a white porcelain cup (about one-third full) and study it in bright sunlight. First, study the color of the urine. Most urine appears orange, yellow or amber at first glance. To truly determine the color of urine, observe the color of the bubbles and the urine at the rim of the container by tilting it.

When the urine characteristics are complex and the physician is not certain of the primary type, he may add certain herbs to the urine and assess its reaction. The way in which the urine reacts to the herbs in terms of the way the herbs settle and spread on the surface of the urine will determine what type of urine it is.

HOW TO EXAMINE THE TONGUE

After examination of the pulse and urine, the tongue should be examined. The tongue is an organ which can tell you about imbalances and disorders of Air, Fire or Water.

FEATURES TO EXAMINE:
- Color
- Deposits of fur or coating
- Dryness
- Presence of pips or pimple-like dots

Air (Lung)Tongue

Color:	Reddish
Dryness:	Dry and rough
Deposits:	Normally clear; sometimes a little fur near the back of the tongue
Pips:	None

Fire (Tripa)Tongue

Color:	Yellowish (especially the fur)
Dryness:	Dry
Deposits:	Yellowish, thick fur over most of the tongue
Pips:	Occasional pips on the sides of the tongue, but generally clear

Water (Bagan)Tongue

Color:	White, pale
Dryness:	Moist and smooth
Deposits:	Thick white fur
Pips:	None

HOW TO EXAMINE THE EYES

Examination of the eyes helps to confirm and support a diagnosis made on the basis of the pulse and urine. However, the individual must be familiar with the natural and inherent color, texture, and fatty deposits present in the eye so as not to confuse them with pathological signs.

Air (lung) Eyes

Air (Lung) eyes tend to be small, with a dry look, especially the eyelashes, which are usually scanty. The eyelids droop, and the whites of the eyes are reddish or may have a muddy look. The eyes may be fixed or very nervous.

Fire (Tripa) Eyes

Fire (Tripa) eyes are generally moderate in size, sharp and lustrous. The lashes are scanty but oily. The black part of the eye may be yellowish, while the white of the eye may be reddish-yellow.

Water (Bagan) Eyes

Water (Bagan) eyes are large and beautiful, moist, with long, thick oily lashes. The eyes are white and pale and may bulge slightly.

5
NUTRITION

INTRODUCTION

The core of maintaining good, consistent health is proper behavior and nutrition. Although nutrition will be discussed in this chapter and behavior in the next, the two are not strictly separate in real life. Understanding nutrition means knowing the type of diet which is most suitable for us, based on our constitutional type, metabolic profile, and immediate health condition. But in addition to being sufficiently familiar with the properties of foods and their combinations to create a healthy diet, we must implement that diet correctly by knowing how much to eat, when to eat, and the role of seasonal variations. In other words, we must be able to change our behavior.

At all times, as we carry out our myriad physical and psychological activities, the balance of the Five Elements in our bodies is forever changing and re-stabilizing. It is by eating or not eating properly, however, that we most directly and dramatically affect this balance.

Failure to obtain enough of the nutrients our bodies need will likely result in disease. A deficiency of a single nutrient may be all it takes, since nutrients act in concert and a deficiency in one may impair the body's ability to use other nutrients even if these others are received in adequate amounts. Even though there is now a constant and abundant supply of most foods, we can easily get into the habit of eating only a small range of foods and never get all the nutrients we need. Our imbalances are perpetuated and disease results.

Fortunately, there are many kinds of foods which, when eaten together, will satisfy all our needs. The nutritional principles outlined below are designed in such a way that, based on your constitutional type [Air (Lung), Fire (Tripa) or Water (Bagan)], you can select food items that will give you the nutrients most likely to be absent in your usual diet because of the propensities of your constitutional type. These Tibetan nutritional principles are very broad guidelines which are effective because they begin with the assumption that people of different constitutional types have different needs and different habit patterns and should therefore eat and do different things. For instance, it is recommended that, in order to receive the necessary supply of protein, a strong Air type should eat mainly animal products, while a strong Fire type should eat dark green vegetables or cereals and grains — *not* animal products.

To make sure you are getting the calories and specific nutrients everyone requires, you may wish to follow the Recommended Dietary Allowance of the U.S. F.D.A. Once you have determined what your requirements are, select your foods based on your current medical condition and the following two categories of guidelines. In the first category are general guidelines that are applicable to everyone, regardless of constitutional type. In the second category are specific guidelines to be applied based on your constitution.

GENERAL GUIDELINES

Taste

Overall, you should like the taste of the food you eat. To do this, you must know how to prepare food in a way that makes it taste good. For instance, let us assume that it has been recommended that you eat more green vegetables. However, you do not enjoy eating raw food; you much prefer spicy food. You can steam your vegetables and add a small amount of pepper. Try to be creative while remaining within the guidelines. It is unfortunate that we do not often use our senses of taste and smell to their full potential.

Eating Habits

In planning a new diet, make sure that you think first about the kinds of foods you eat consistently and those that you grew up eating. Your whole metabolic system has been conditioned by these kinds of foods. Any sudden or drastic change in diet can cause an upset in the metabolic system which in turn can make it very difficult for the new healthy diet to be metabolized properly. Whenever you make a change, particularly a drastic one such as eliminating all animal products from your diet, do it gradually, over a period of one to three months depending on your condition. Also, do it carefully, watching for changes in your metabolic rate and eliminative functions. If you notice any changes, consider slowing down the rate of change in your diet.

Digestive Ability

If you have poor digestive power, then no matter how nutritious the content of your food, it will not be digested completely and provide the body with nourishment. It is therefore very important to assess your digestive power before starting a new diet and to watch for any improvement after you start the diet. For about two weeks before beginning any new diet, and for about the same period of time after starting, keep a record of some of the signs noticeable in your digestive tract. For example: Do you feel energetic or sluggish after eating? Does your stomach feel comfortable, or full and heavy? Do you have gas, rumbling sounds, loose stools or constipation? If you notice signs of improvement, then this indicates that the new diet is working and your digestive power is probably fine. If you discover no improvement, this indicates that your digestive power is weak and must first be strengthened before changing to a new diet. A simple way to improve minor digestive weakness is by drinking a cup of ginger tea after meals and by increasing your amount of exercise — by jogging, for instance. This combination of ginger and exercise can improve digestive power in about a month. For more severe weakness, herbal stimulants such as pomegranate pills are recommended.

Eliminative Functions

If you find that certain foods consistently cause constipation, diarrhea, or a disruption of your bowel movements, it usually means that this food should not be part of your diet. For a healthy person, one or two bowel movements per day are essential. It is preferable to have a bowel movement in the morning when you first get up. To regulate yourself, drink a glass of cold water upon awakening. You will find within ten days that you will have a regular bowel movement in the morning.

Eating Practices

Since it takes about twenty minutes after food reaches your stomach for the brain to receive the message that food has been eaten, it is best to eat slowly. Allow at least twenty minutes to eat a meal.

Eat regularly spaced meals to avoid hunger or binges of over-eating.

Cut your food into small, easily digestible pieces, and pay attention to the taste, smell and texture of your food. Avoid doing anything that distracts you, like watching television or reading.

When you are feeling stress or are in an emotional mood, try not to eat. Instead, try some other interesting activity such as taking an herbal bath or talking to a friend.

THE THREE PROPERTIES OF FOOD

Types of food are differentiated on the basis of three properties called **taste, potency,** and **quality.** Each of these properties has a different therapeutic effect on the body.

Tastes

There are six tastes: sweet, sour, salty, pungent, bitter and astringent. Sweet refers primarily to starches and sugars. Sour refers to fermented or acidic food, and salty refers to alkalis and regular table salt. Pungent is the same as spicy and acrid. Bitter is the taste of bitter herbs like gentian or senna leaves. Astringent has a neutral taste but includes herbs such as witch hazel and alum, which have a constricting effect on the tongue. The six tastes are derived from the following combinations of the five elements:

$$
\begin{array}{rcl}
\text{Earth} + \text{Water} &=& \text{Sweet} \\
\text{Fire} + \text{Earth} &=& \text{Sour} \\
\text{Water} + \text{Fire} &=& \text{Salty} \\
\text{Fire} + \text{Air} &=& \text{Pungent} \\
\text{Air} + \text{Space} &=& \text{Bitter} \\
\text{Earth} + \text{Air} &=& \text{Astringent}
\end{array}
$$

THERAPEUTIC ACTIONS OF THE SIX TASTES

Taste	Air (Lung)	Fire (Tripa)	Water (Bagan)
Bitter	Increases	Decreases	Decreases
Pungent	Increases	Increases	Decreases
Astringent	Increases	Decreases	Decreases
Sour	Decreases	Increases	Increases
Salty	Decreases	Increases	Increases
Sweet	Decreases	Decreases	Increases

Potency

The potency of food or herbs is determined by whether it cools or heats the body when digested. The body requires both heating and cooling to allow the metabolic process to function efficiently. The potency of the foods/herbs we eat allows us to harmonize with environmental or seasonal changes.

In general, foods/herbs with a cooling potency have either a sweet, bitter or astringent taste. Likewise foods/herbs with a heating potency have either a pungent, sour or salty taste.

TASTES — POTENCIES AND EFFECTS

E=Earth   W=Water   F=Fire

E+W=Sweet		F+E=Sour		F+W=Salty		W+Wind=Bitter		F+Wind=Hot		E+Wind=Astringent	
heavy	10	hot	7	oily	4	cool	9	light	9	cold	4
blunt	7	dry	6	coarse	4	moist	5	coarse	7	blunt	4
cool	5	oily	4	sharp	3	blunt	3	cry	6	dry	2
moist	5	compact	4	hot	2	coarse	3	mobile	6		
compact	5	heavy	3	heavy	1	light	2	sharp	6		
oily	4	sharp	2	dry	1	soft	1	hot	3		
smooth	3	coarse	1	soft	1	mobile	5				
soft	1			mobile	1						

THE TWENTY ATTRIBUTES AND QUALITIES

The twenty attributes may be divided into ten pairs of opposites (i.e. hot and cold, wet and dry, etc.) which are the positive and negative manifestations of all forces in the universe (see Chapter 2). They constitute the fundamental nature of all objects both animate and inanimate.

Generally, the cold, wet, heavy, gross or yin qualities go together, as do the hot, dry, light, subtle or yang qualities. Yin or cold qualities tend to descend and contract and stabilize the physical part of the individual, while the yang or hot qualities ascend and expand and create vitality and consciousness.

We see the pairs of opposites at work all around us in our day to day experiences and in the objects with which we come into contact. Though similar qualities produce corresponding results — i.e. a cold, drying diet will cause increased Lung just as a cold, dry emotional attitude will do the same — we are in real life constantly in the middle of the two pairs of opposites, and trying to find our place seems to be the immediate problem. Our life and environment has become so complex that it is no longer entirely possible to work on each extreme by applying the opposite attribute, like heat in cold weather or cold packs during fever. It is in light of this that we should carefully consider our constitutional typology in relationship to any immediate health imbalance.

The twenty attributes may be subsumed into four major categories which are dry or moist, heavy or light. These four are particularly helpful in determining dietary and herbal treatment for the Three Nepas. For instance, since the main quality of Air (Lung) is dryness while that of Water (Bagan) is moisture, herbs and foods which are drying (bitter, pungent and astringent) increase Air (Lung) and decrease Water (Bagan). Those that are moistening (sweet, salty and sour) increase Water (Bagan) and decrease Air (Lung).

The qualities of lightness and heaviness of herbs and foods tend to increase lightness or heaviness in the body. Heavy qualities of herbs such as sweet, salty and astringent tend to promote weight and firmness in the body while bitter, pungent and sour are light and cause loss of weight, yet have a strong capacity to digest well.

The use of foods and herbs is determined by their taste and potency. Taste is determined by power and qualities of the food or herb. The eight characteristics or potencies of a food or drug are:

heavy
oily
cool
blunt
light
coarse or rough
hot or pungent
sharp

Heavy, oily, cool and blunt foods or herbs are therapeutic for Air (Lung) and Fire (Tripa) disorders, while light, rough, pungent and sharp are therapeutic for treating Water (Bagan) disorders.

These eight potencies play an important role in blancing nature, or in neutralizing or detoxifying imbalances in the body. For instance, disorders with light, coarse, cool characteristics are neutralized and eliminated by food and herbs with heavy, oily and pungent qualities.

The essence of all qualities and potencies may be subsumed into hot and cold power. The eight potencies consist of seventeen qualities and are classified according to qualitative and quantitative characteristics and functions. One may assign arbitrary units (1 through 10) in order to designate the predominance of herb qualities and quantities. The five basic elements which compose a molecule are earth, water, fire, air and space particles. Combinations of these particles give rise to molecular structures which then form into structures which have more differentiated qualities and functions. The qualities of earth are heaviness, bluntness, smoothness, oiliness and softness. Fire is pungent, sharp, dry, coarse, light, oily and mobile. Air is light, mobile, cold, coarse, and dry. Water is cool, liquid, cohesive, soft and subtle. Space is dry, light mobile, clear and formless

The six major tastes are composed of the following qualities. Salty, astringent, and sweet tastes are essentially heavy. Salty, sour, oily tastes are essentially oily. Astringent, bittter, and sweet are essentially cool.

Note the tables below. Observe the relationship among the qualitative units of the tastes. Sour has more heavy units than sweet. Salty has more oily units than sour. By studying the table, one can observe the difference in composition in a food or herb.

In order to balance the application of herbs or diet in treating disorders, it is first important to understand that disorders may also be described in terms of qualities. There are twenty qualities or characteristics in relationship to disorders. They are listed in the tables below in relationship to the seventeen therapeutic qualities of food and herbs.

QUALITIES IN RELATIONSHIP TO DISORDERS

Compound	Principal	Secondary	Remedies
Double	Sweet	+ Sour	triple combined disorders
Triple	Sweet	+ Sour+Salty	triple predominance of phlegm and bile
Quadruple	Sweet	+ Sour+Bitter+Salty	triple with predominance of wind

Composition	Interaction	Composition	Product
4 cold Wind/u	+	2 Earth/u	= 4 cold units
4 blunt Earth/u	+	2 Wind/u	= 4 cold units
1 dry Earth/u	+	1 dry Wind/u	= 2 dry units
6 heavy Earth/u	+	4 heavy Water/u	= 10 heavy units
4 blunt Earth/u	+	3 blunt Water/u	= 7 blunt units
No compostion		5 cold Water/u	= 5 cool units
1 dry Earth/u	-	6 moist Water/u	= 5 moist units
5 compact Earth/u		No composition	= 5 compact units

PROPERTIES AND THERAPEUTIC QUALITIES

Based on a thorough understanding of the mechanisms set forth in the tables above, one can prepare different compounds of food and herbs to treat disorders more effectively. Listed below are a few different preparations of compounds of herbs and food for the treatment of corresponding disorders. Multiple combinations are used to treat complex disorders and there may be as many as two to six major multiple combinations of herbs or food.

For instance, you can take pomegranate in conjunction with other herbs in treating abdominal disorders. The principal taste of pomegranate is sour and sweet. Consequently, its physical composition is earth and water. Its qualitative composition is sweetness, i.e. heavy, blunt, cool, moist, stable, oily, smooth and soft. Its quantitative composition is as follows, in terms of arbitrary units:

| 10 heavy units | 7 blunt units | 5 cool units | 5 moist units |
| 5 stable units | 4 oily units | 3 smooth units | 1 soft unit |

Increasing reaction occurs when both reacting elements have similar qualities. Decreasing reaction occurs when the reacting elements have opposite qualities. For instance, one of the six moist water units neutralizes the one dry earth unit, resulting in five moist units. In the case of the five cool water units, they are retained because earth does not contain any corresponding reacting units.

SEASONAL VARIATIONS

When you are planning a diet, the time of the year should influence both how much you eat and what you eat. For example, during the summer, a time when the heat causes a loss of body fluid and energy, foods that are cooling and moist are preferable. However, since digestive power is reduced during summer, smaller amounts of food are necessary.

SEASONAL VARIATIONS				
Season	Elements	Taste	Potencies	Relative Body Strength
Late Winter	Fire & Air ↑ Water & Earth ↓	Pungent	Sharp & Hot ↑ Cool & Oily ↓	Strong
Spring	Fire & Earth ↑ Water ↓	Astringent	Sharp & Dry ↑ Cool ↓	Weak
Early Summer	Earth & Air ↑ Fire ↓	Bitter	Dry & Hot ↑	Weaker
Late Summer	Earth & Fire ↑	Sour	Heavy ↑	Weak
Autumn	Fire & Water ↑	Salty	Heavy ↑	Stronger
Early Winter	Earth & Water ↑	Sweet	Heavy & Cool ↑	Very Strong

Healthy Foods and Activities for the Six Seasons

LATE WINTER (January–February)

Eat foods that are hot, salty, sour or sweet. Fresh or clarified butter, milk, wine, jaggery, and foods high in protein such as rich meaty soups are particularly good at this time.

Keep warm and sun yourself often. Apply sesame oil after bathing.

SPRING (March–April)

Eat foods that are hot, bitter, pungent or astringent. Celery, ginger, hot peppers, non-oily herbs and spicy foods in general are good at this time. Replace heavy, oily meats with lighter and dryer foods, with grains left for a year or the aged meat of animals living in dry areas, such as mountain goats. Liquids should favor honey and ginger tea after meals.

Wash with lentil powder instead of soap. Perfume yourself with a flower scent.

SUMMER (May–June)

Eat foods that are sweet in taste, cooling in potency, light and oily in quality. Avoid salty, hot and sour foods. Drink lots of liquids. Beer is permissible, with ice.

Keep cool by wearing light clothing, opening windows, bathing with lukewarm water, and staying out of the sun. Burn sandalwood incense.

LATE SUMMER (July–August)

Eat foods that are sour, salty or sweet. Light, warming, and oily foods can also be eaten. Liquids such as beer and wine made from grains grown in dry areas are fine.

Avoid excess cold at this time.

AUTUMN (September–October)

Eat foods that are sweet, bitter, or astringent.

Perfume yourself with a cooling fragrance.

EARLY WINTER (November–December)

Eat foods that are pungent, salty or sour.

Keep warm, but avoid getting too much heat.

SPECIFIC GUIDELINES
Planning a Diet for Air (Lung) Constitutional Profile

Since Air (Lung) constitutional individuals tend to be basically cold, dry, light and mobile in terms of physiological and biological functions and characteristics, a diet which is warming, moistening and nourishing contains the qualities which are most therapeutic. Foods that are sweet, sour and salty have these qualities.

In general, a hearty diet of protein, rich and high-carbohydrate foods is most important for Air types. Three regular meals a day are recommended, with breakfast being the most important and lunch the least important. Severe fasting should not be undertaken, nor should any meals be missed, especially during stressful times.

Breakfast and dinner should consist of well-cooked food only, and should be eaten warm. For example, breakfast cereals should be eaten with warm milk and bread should be toasted. Grains, cereals, and animal products in particular should be well-cooked and eaten with a soup or broth to help digestion. Raw foods should be avoided; vegetables, for example, should be steamed.

Breakfast might include grape juice, oatmeal with heated milk, toast with clarified butter and sesame seeds, or sauteed tofu with jaggery juice.

Lunch might include chicken soup, dark green vegetables such as spinach, cucumber or okra sauteed in olive oil, well-cooked and mildly seasoned beans such as black lentils or mung cooked with mild spices, or brown rice cooked with ginger and jaggery.

Dinner might include split pea soup, fish or well-cooked chicken sauteed with vegetables in clarified butter, wheat bulgur seasoned with mild spices and yogurt.

When one of the four primary characteristics of the Lung constitution is predominant in an individual, foods which are normally not suitable for Air may be recommended until the characteristic is back in balance. For instance, if the cold quality predominates, foods that are pungent and drying may be

temporarily helpful. But if dry and light characteristics pre-
dominate, then under no circumstances should pungent and
dry foods be recommended. Rather, more heavy, oily and
moistening food such as sesame oil, avocadoes, meat, rich
grains etc. should be recommended.

Planning a Diet for Fire (Tripa) Constitutional Profile

The Fire (Tripa) constitutional type is predominantly hot
in terms of its physiological and biological characteristics.
Therefore foods with cooling or heat-dispelling characteristics
are recommended. Foods that taste sweet, astringent and bitter
are cooling in nature and thus therapeutic for Fire types. Of
those three tastes, bitter foods such as vegetables and bitter
fruits are highly recommended for Fire diets.

Generally, a diet which is rich in vegetables, fruits, cereals
and grains is most beneficial for Fire types. The consumption
of meat should be avoided except for occasional fish and white
meats, as should fermented foods like blue cheese, wine or
vinegar. In general, foods with a pungent or sour taste or a
heating quality should be minimized and those with a cooling
quality increased. Vegetables and fruits should be eaten raw
as often as possible. The digestive power of the Fire person is
usually very great, so he must always watch for signs of excess
bile like an upset stomach or excessive gas. Unlike an Air
(Lung) person, he does not require three regular meals a day,
so he should eat only when he feels hungry.

Breakfast might include fresh fruit juice, an apple, a slice
of melon, or wheat bread.

Lunch might include a salad of light green vegetable, apple
juice, or oat bread.

Dinner may be chicken or fish cooked with a little turmeric,
cumin and coriander, white rice, vegetable soup or salad.

Planning a Diet for Water (Bagan) Constitutional Profile

The Water (Bagan) constitutional type is predominantly
cold, moist, slow and heavy in terms of physiological

characteristics. Therefore, foods that have warming, drying, lightening and stimulating qualities are recommended. Foods that taste pungent, bitter and astringent — particularly pungent — are highly therapeutic for Water. In general, fasting and a light diet are an essential part of any dietary plan for Water types in order to balance the excess of the mucus and body fat.

Light and easily digestible foods are generally best for a Water type. Raw, unripe and cold foods should not be eaten. Foods should be well cooked, eaten warm and cut into easily digestible pieces. Grains and cereals should be cooked using herbs with a heating quality. Lunch is the most important meal. In fact, just two meals a day is optimum, or breakfast and dinner can simply be vegetable juice or something very light.

Breakfast might consist of hot herbal tea with ginger, cinnamon, and honey.

Lunch might include light green vegetables sauteed in vegetable oil with pungent spices, brocolli, okra and radish soup, or millet cooked with jaggery and ginger.

Dinner might include brown rice cooked with garlic, ginger and honey.

DIETARY GUIDELINES FOR THE THREE TYPES

	Air (Lung)		
	Recommended	Occasional	Not Recommended
Animal Products	poultry	rabbit	goat
	fish	duck	pork
	eggs	fresh dried meat	
	old goat butter	fresh butter	
	old cow's butter	fresh cow's milk	
	butter of sheep	beef	
	cow's cheese	mutton	
	cow's whey	yogurt	
	old ghee		

AIR (Lung)

	Recommended	Occasional	Not Recommended
Grains	wheat millet white basmati brown rice cooked oats barley amaranth quinoa	corn	dry oats buckwheat white bread regular white rice
	(Grain should be 35–45% of diet)		
Legumes	tofu dahl brown lentils aduki black beans garbanzo soy beans tempeh pintos anasazi mung kidney lima chana	none	split peas Chinese red beans red lentils
Vegetables	(cooked only) carrots brocolli winter squashes spinach angelica root turloulis tomato red cabbage peas potatoes sweet potatoes corn onions sea vegetables globe artichoke cilantro arrowroot	(cooked only) lettuce green pepper hot peppers egg plants mushrooms kale turnip collard greens ginger parsnips beets brussel sprouts mustard greens	raw cabbage raw lettuce light green veg., especially raw burdock dandelion bok choy
	(Vegetables should be 25–30% of the diet)		

AIR (Lung)

	Recommended	Occasional	Not Recommended
Nuts & Seeds	linseeds walnuts sesame sun flower flax seed cashew pumpkin	coconut almond hazelnut chestnuts	
Fruits	(room temp.) bananas oranges grapefruits apples pineapples	peaches plum grapes strawberry pear blueberry cherry	cranberry lemon dried fruits watermelon cantaloupe apricot
Oils, Salts & Condiments	old butter sesame oil peanut oil ghee olive oil miso tamari rock, read, black & sea salt umebashi ginger butter garlic butter	sunflower oil corn oil safflower oil	mustard oil
Beverages	cow's milk wine	wine	cold water coffee black tea hard liquor

AIR (Lung)

	Recommended	Occasional	Not Recommended
Herbs & Spices	angelica anise asfoetida cardamon cinnamon fenugreek clove cumin aquilaria heat (eagel wood) fennel garlic - heat ginger jaggery nutmeg onion sesame stinging nettle solomon seal terminalia chebula	chili coriander shatavari pippali	

LUNG—KRIPA (Vata—Pitta)

	Recommended
Animal Products	poultry rabbit fish eggs butter cow's milk
Grains	wheat millet white basmati brown rice cooked oats barley amaranth quinoa

(Grain should be 35–45% of diet)

AIR—FIRE (Lung—Tripa)

Recommended

Legumes   tofu
brown lentils
dahl
aduki
black beans
anasazi
garbanzo
kidney
mung
pinto
lima
tempeh
chana

Vegetables   (steamed or raw)
carrot
broccoli
squashes
spinach
tomato
red cabbage
peas
potatoes
sweet potatoes
corn
onion
sea vegetables
bell pepper
cilantro
globe artichoke
angelica
beets
arrowroot
    (Vegetables should be 25–30% of the diet)

AIR—FIRE (Lung—Tripa)

	Recommended
Nuts & Seeds	linseed walnut sesame sunflower flax cashew pumpkin
Fruits	banana orange grapefruit apple pineapple strawberry blueberry cherry plum
Oils, Salts & Condiments	ginger butter garlic butter sesame oil peanut oil olive oil ghee sunflower oil safflower oil corn oil rock, red, black, sea salt tamari miso
Beverages	cow's milk

AIR—FIRE (Lung—Tripa)

	Recommended
Herbs &	coriander
Spices	anise
	fenugreek
	clove
	cumin
	aquilaria
	fennel
	ginger
	jaggery
	nutmeg
	onion
	sesame
	solomon seal
	terminalia
	chebula
	cinnamon
	coriander

FIRE (Tripa)

	Recommended	Occasional	Not Recommended
Animal	rabbit	pork	poultry
Products	fresh ghee	skim cow's milk	fish
	goat's milk	fresh goat butter	beef
	cow's milk	fresh cow butter	lamb
	(most herbivo-	new butter	mutton
	rous animals)		shellfish
	(*note: if hot Fire		
	one should not		
	have any animal		
	products)		

(Generally, animal products should be kept to minimum)

Grains	white basmati	oats	rye
	white noodles	barley (toasted)	brown rice
	millet		amaranth
	wheat		
	corn		
	quinoa		
	tapioca		
	regular white rice		
	buckwheat		

(Grains should be 25% of the diet)

FIRE (Tripa)

	Recommended	Occasional	Not Recommended
Legumes	adzukis	tofu	tempeh
	anasazi	lima	soy beans
	black beans	chana	redlentils
	garbanzos		Chinese red beans
	kidneys		
	pintos		
	mung		
	dahl		
	brown lentils		
Vegetables	zucchini	raw spinach	ginger
	cucumber	charbl	radish
	yam	sea vegetables	avocado
	brocolli	bell pepper	garlic
	cabbage	potatoes	tomato
	cauliflower	jerusalem	eggplant
	lettuce	artichokes	chilis
	kale	rutabaga	hot peppers
	winter squashes	sweet corn	mustard greens
	celery	cilantro	onions
	burdock	beets	sauerkraut
	peas		globe artichokes
	green beans		water chesnut
	asparagus		bamboo shoots
	carrot		turnip
	bok choy		mushrooms
	potatoes		
	spinach		
	red cabbage		
	turnip greens		
	parsley		
	collard greens		
	dandelion		
	parsnip		
	brussel sprouts		

(Vegetables should be 50% of the diet)

FIRE (Tripa)

	Recommended	Occasional	Not Recommended
Nuts & Seeds	none	sunflower seed pumpkin seed	hazelnut walnut chestnut cashew flax seed sesame seed peanut almonds coconut
Fruits	melons cantaloupe barberry peaches pears	grape grapefruit apples pineapple strawberry plums raisins blueberry cherry banana	lemon lime apricot cranberry
Oils, Salts & Condiments	ghee fresh butter	sunflower oil corn oil safflower oil sea salt	butter mustard oil sesame oil peanut oil olive oil black & red salt temari miso
Beverages	water	skimmed milk	wine cow's milk coffee black tea beer hard liquor

FIRE (Tripa)

	Recommended	Occasional	Not Recommended
Herbs & Spices	barberry (cooling) cucumber seed (c) dandelion (c) ephedra (warming) gentian (c) gotu kola (c) guggul (c) (Indian bedelium) hibiscus (c) licorice (neutral) shilagit (w) white sandalwood(c) red sandalwood (for blood) (c) safflower (c) saffron (cooling for blood — Fire) shatavari (c) raisins (c) rhododendron (c) rose macrophyil (red) (n) rose sericea (yellow) (c) tumeric (c) terminalia chebula (n) terminalia belarica (n)	cinnamon coriandor	

FIRE—WATER (Tripa—Bagan)

	Recommended
Animal Products	goat meat rabbit ghee goat's milk cow's milk

(Generally, animal products should be kept to a minimum)

FIRE—WATER (Tripa—Bagan)

Recommended

Grains   white basmati
white noodles
millet
wheat
barley
corn
quinoa
tapioca
(Grains should be 25% of the diet)

Legumes   aduki
andsazi
black beans
garbanzo
kidneys
pintos
mung
dahl
brown lentils
chana

FIRE—WATER (Tripa—Bagan)

	Recommended
Vegetables	zucchini
	cucumber
	yam
	broccoli
	cabbage
	cauliflower
	lettuce
	kale
	winter squashes
	celery
	burdock
	peas
	green beans
	asparagus
	carrot
	bok choy
	potatoes
	spinach
	red cabbage
	turnip greens
	parsley
	collard greens
	dandelion greens
	parsnips
	brussel sprouts
	cilantro
Nuts & Seeds	sunflower seed
	pumpkin seed
Fruits	melon
	cantaloupe
	barberry
	peaches
	pears
	grape
	strawberry
Oils, Salts & Condiments	ghee
	fresh butter
	sunflower oil
	no salt

FIRE—WATER (Tripa—Bagan)

	Recommended
Beverages	water
Herbs & Spices	licorice
	raisins
	terminalia
	belerica
	embilica offinalis
	gotu kola
	guggul
	hibiscus
	shilagit
	red sandelwood
	safflower
	shatavari
	raisins
	red rose
	yellow rose
	turmeric
	terminalia
	chebula

WATER (Bagan)

	Recommended	Occasional	Not Recommended
Animal Products	rabbit (flesh from lower part of male & upper part of female)	yogurt	goat
		fresh cheese	pork
		sheep/mutton, boiled with asfoetida, ginger & whey	frozen, roasted, uncooked meat
	fish		beef
	poultry		
	old dried meat		
	old butter of sheep		
	cow's cheese		
	one-year old butter of cow or goat		
	other herbivourous animals		

WATER (Bagan)

	Recommended	Occasional	Not Recommended

Grains	white basmati
	cooked oats
	dry oats
	toasted/cooked
	  barley
		wheat
		brown rice—
		  with ginger
		  & gur
		regular white
		  rice
		toasted millet
		buckwheat—
		  one year old
			fresh buckwheat
			corn

(Grains should be 20–25% of diet)

	Recommended	Occasional	Not Recommended
Legumes	split peas dahl	mung brown lentils chana	tofu kidney bean soy bean pintos aduki anasazi garbanzo lima red lentils chinese red beans

	Recommended	Occasional	Not Recommended
Vegetables	(cooked only) onion garlic young radish daikon mushrooms cooked tomato hot pepper green pepper chili's turnips rutabaga angelica sorrel leaves Himalayan rhubarb bamboo shoots celery	(cooked only) eggplant sauerkraut water chestnut lettuce spinach globe artichoke cilantro burdock dandelion parsnip bok choy cabbage cauliflower mustard greens arrowroot	raw vegetables potato sweet potato cucumber squashes peas green beans kale collards beets broccoli brussel sprouts

(Vegetables should be 35% of the diet)

WATER (Bagan)

	Recommended	Occasional	Not Recommended
Nuts & Seeds	none	sunflower seed pumpkin seed sesame seed	walnut cashew chestnut flax linseed hazel nut almonds peanuts coconut
Fruits	pomegranite raisins tamarind	grapes orange lemon lime strawberry pears peaches	plums apricots blueberry cherry pineapple melons cantaloupe banana
Oils, Salts & Condiments	safflower oil black salt	peanut oil sesame oil sunflower oil ghee tamari old butter	fats corn oil olive oil mustard oil sea salt miso
Beverages	beer	wine boiled water cow's milk coffee black tea	cold water hard liquor

WATER (Bagan)

	Recommended	Occasional	Not Recommended
Herbs & Spices	asfoetida ashwaganda black pepper chili cardamon cinnamon clove cumin fennel fenugreek garlic ginger licorice sesame raisins pippali	Tumeric	

AIR—WATER (Lung—Bagan)

	Recommended
Animal Products	poultry fish (both cooked with brown sesame seeds) fresh & old dried meat cheese yoghurt beef, boiled with asfoetida, ginger & black salt
Grains	white basmati cooked oats dry oats toasted millet barley (Grains should be 20—25% of diet)
Legumes	split peas dhal

AIR—WATER (Lung—Bagan)

Recommended

Vegetables (cooked only)
onion
garlic
ginger
radish
diakon
mushrooms
cooked tomato
bamboo shoots
globe artichoke
celery
hot peppers
bell peppers
turnips
rutabaga
eggplant
lettuce
turnip
mustard green
parsnip
        (Vegetables should be 35% of the diet)

Nuts &   none
Seeds

Fruits   pomegranite
raisin
tamarind
peach
pear
strawberry
grapes

Oils, Salts   safflower oil
&Condi-   sunflower oil
ments   black salt

Beverages   none

AIR—WATER (Lung—Bagan)

	Recommended
Herbs & **Spices**	angelica
	asfoetida
	cardamon
	cinnamon
	clove
	cumin
	fennel
	fenugreek
	garlic
	ginger
	sesame
	ashwaganda
	black pepper

6
BEHAVIOR

Healthy behavior begins by considering the goals, both short-term and long-term, of your health plan. Tibetan medicine distinguishes three such goals: increased life span, increased enjoyment, and increased fulfillment of spiritual needs.

HOW TO INCREASE YOUR LIFE SPAN

To live a long life, you must have a balanced mind, body and spirit. To maintain this balance over a long period of time requires an awareness of how you fit into the natural harmony of the environment. By consciously attempting to enhance the equilibrium among your organs and body systems, your emotions and attitudes, and your relations with others, you can increase this type of awareness. Following is a list of recommendations on how to increase your life span:

Take every precaution to protect yourself from known danger; try to live in a safe area.

Live with a knowledge of your constitutional type and follow the suggested eating habits, behavior, etc.

Get plenty of sleep. Do not try to make up for lost sleep by sleeping at odd hours; instead, take it easy and make it up the next night during your normal sleep period. Air types can take short naps during the afternoon but other types should refrain from this habit. Water types can fast or undergo pancha karma (see Chapter 7) if they find that they are sleeping too much or feeling too lethargic.

Keep sexual activities responsible. Sex with a partner who is ill or undergoing severe emotional distress is not recommended. Sex during pregnancy and menstrual periods should be avoided. Sexual acts such as adultery and bestiality are always harmful.

Make exercise part of your routine. Water types should include regular strenuous exercise in their lives, though for Air types light, relaxing exercise is better. Fire types should not over-exercise or be too competitive and should try to make their exercise enjoyable.

Practice good hygiene and bathe regularly. Normally, a bath should be in lukewarm to warm water, not too hot, since this may cause skin problems and hair loss. Hot mineral spring baths are best taken in the spring and autumn.

Apply oil to your body and do self-massage. This is especially beneficial for Air types. They should rub heated sesame oil on the crown of the head, vertebrae, sternum, palms, heels and in the ears, especially before bedtime.

Maintain a high ethical standard. For example, keep promises you have made and keep secrets others have entrusted to you so that you develop trust and responsibility. Also, try to get to the truth in all situations and do not depend upon the advice of those whom you do not consider to be truthful.

Treat people fairly, patiently and respectfully, and try to resolve enmity whenever possible. Show special respect to those who have helped you, your parents, and the elderly.

FOLLOWING YOUR NATURAL URGES

There are thirteen natural urges which, if suppressed, may contribute to poor health. The following is a list of these suppressed urges, including their symptoms and simple remedies.

1. The symptoms of **suppressed hunger** are physical weakness, dizziness and difficulty in swallowing. The remedy is to begin by eating small quantities of light, oily and warm foods. Slowly increase the quantity as your body gets used to it. Do not eat large quantities immediately. You may wish to try:

- a rich broth created by making a rice soup with ghee, meat soup (do not eat the meat, however; just the soup), and light cheese
- a light grain soup prepared in a similar manner

2. The symptoms of **suppressed thirst** are dizziness, palpitation, and mental dullness. The remedy is cooling foods that are sweet in taste, or:

- sprinkling cold water on the body and face if one feels weak and dizzy
- drinking cold curd
- drinking cold fruit and vegetable juices

3. The symptoms of **suppressed vomiting** are swelling, sores, itching, eyestrain, and flu. The remedies are fasting, inhalation of aquilaria and sandalwood incenses, eating food in more liquid form in small quantities, and drinking water with a small amount of honey.

4. The symptoms of **suppressed sneezing** are a lack of sensory and mental clarity, dizziness, a stiff neck and a loss of sensitivity in the face. The remedies are:

- nasaya, a nasal treatment comprised of taking a pinch of nutmeg and asafoetida powder and mixing it with 15 drops of clarified butter mixed with a pinch of honey
- inhalation of aquilaria and sandalwood incenses
- repeated gazing at the sun

5. The symptoms of **suppressed yawning** are tremors, numbness, convulsions and insomnia. The remedy may follow the same treatment as that for suppressed sneezing, as well as eating nourishing foods high in complex carbohydrates and foods or herbs which reduce Air (Lung) conditions generally.

6. The symptoms of **suppressed breathing** are shortness of breath and pains in the upper chest. The remedies are breathing exercises and plenty of rest for your mind, body and speech. Diet, behavior and therapies which treat Lung disorders in general are highly effective.

7. The symptoms of **suppressed sleep** are lethargy, dullness, heaviness, dimness of vision, and difficulty in digestion. The remedies are:

- massage the body — especially the head, palms, soles of the feet and the ears — with heated sesame oil, then make an effort to sleep
- drink hot milk or eat soup with nutmeg
- take a nutritive and nourishing soup of chicken or sheep
- fresh, mild wine

8. The symptoms of **suppressed mucus** are breathing problems, congestion, hiccups, and pressure on the heart. The remedy is pancha karma (see Chapter 7), particularly emetics. One may also prepare a mucus-expelling remedy of equal portions ginger, brown sugar, and Indian long pepper, the mixture to be boiled in a cup of water and taken when only a third of the water remains.

9. The symptoms of **suppressed saliva** are sneezing, head colds, and flu. The remedy is to rest and gargle, to drink light, fresh wine, to sleep regularly, and to enjoy pleasant and stress-reducing conversations with friends during one's leisure time.

10. The symptoms of **suppressed flatus** are constipation and intestinal cramps. The remedy is a purgative.

11 and 12. The symptoms of **suppressed bowel movements and/or urination** are pain and irritation during eventual evacuation or urination. The two problems are treated in a similar manner since in both cases the disorder involves the reflux of the descending Lung. The remedies are:

- herbal purgatives
- enemas
- after an herbal steaming with ginger, bay and eucalyptus leaves, heated sesame oil is applied all over the body, especially the back and front of the midsection
- heated packs of sesame oil are tightly wrapped around the lower back and constantly heated with a hot water bottle
- the lower back is wrapped with animal skin during the daytime
- a special herbal preparation known as Ba-sam sMan-mar is orally taken on a regular basis (see Biodata at end of book for ordering herbs)

13. The symptom of **suppressed emission of semen** is a loss of sexual energy. The remedies are:

- as above, i.e. the application of heated sesame oil packs, followed by the animal skin wrapping and the ingestion of Ba-sam sMan-mar
- gradual sexual activity after the above treatment
- nourishing and nutritious food such as clarified butter, milk, white meat, and rich nutritious wine all help to increase semen quality
- medicated herbal baths, nutritious soups and herbs generally

STRESS REDUCTION

We continually experience stress from many sources: our bodies and thoughts, the people we encounter, and the environment and climate in which we live. Though we may detest the noise and crowds of the city or the icy cold of winter, we usually learn to face these kinds of stress. The demands on our time made by others and various threats to our security are often harder to accept, and consequently the level of our stress shoots higher. Still more stressful may be the changes that often go unnoticed in our bodies, such as during illness, loss of sleep, or pregnancy. However, even more stress can be produced by our own thoughts, as when we label our experiences rather than face the truth, or when we hold in our emotions rather than experience our feelings.

When we are healthy we know when it is time to relax, to escape; we do something directly in order to reduce the mounting stress. When we are unhealthy we let stress mount until our system breaks down completely. Each person has a different reaction and tolerance for stress, but it is greatly determined by his or her constitutional type. Following is a list of symptoms of excessive stress in each of the three types. It is important to remember that many of the symptoms of stress listed here are also present when there are imbalances caused by other factors.

For Air (Lung) types, symptoms of stress are:

muscular tension	diffused pain	dizziness
tension headaches	palpitations	fatigue
cold extremities	frequent sighing	disturbed sleep
gas and bloating	constipation	cracking joints
dry skin	ringing in ears	goose pimples
menstrual problems	anxiety	nervousness
distraction	compulsiveness	

For Fire (Tripa) types, symptoms of stress are:

headaches	liver pains	afternoon fatigue
diarrhea	nausea	appetite loss
anger	irritability	anxiety
bitter taste in mouth after waking		

For Water (Bagan) types, symptoms of stress are:

lethargy	dullness	heaviness
cold extremities	kidney pains	procrastination
poor digestion	obesity	frequent urination
discomfort after eating	resistance to change	

WAYS TO DEAL WITH STRESS AND STRAIN

In order to deal with the signs and symptoms that occur due to stress and strain in relation to one's constitutional typology, a number of techniques covering the entire range of the individual's experience and behavior are recommended. These techniques are comprised of:

- Environmental and Behavioral Changes
- Bodywork and Acupressure
- Meditation

AIR (LUNG) CONSTITUTIONAL TYPES

ENVIRONMENTAL AND BEHAVIORAL CHANGES
The following lifestyle patterns are recommended:
- Get eight hours of sleep. If you get less, try to make it up with a thirty-minute nap after lunch.
- Avoid very strenuous and stressful activities on an empty stomach.
- Avoid having an empty stomach for long periods of time.
- Avoid strenuous exercises. Instead, practice light, relaxing exercises such as walking or T'ai Ch'i and progress from these to more strenuous exercises.

- Avoid prolonged exposure to cold and breezes.
- Avoid great heights such as mountain tops, or even high-rise buildings.
- Avoid cool, dry climates.
- Keep the skin moist and healthy. It is a sensitive organ, especially for Lung types.
- Keep your home and workplace cozy, warm, and dimly lit. Do not use bright lights.
- Avoid noisy places and aggressive, unpleasant people.
- Work and link up with like-minded people.
- Avoid the early morning hours.
- Dark blue is the most therapeutic color.
- Always find time to relax with a hot bath, massage and music after a long day's work.

BODYWORK AND ACUPRESSURE
Bodywork

Apply heated sesame or aquilaria oil on the entire body and massage the entire body, particularly the tensed areas. The best time to do this is before bed; if possible, leave the oil on the body for the night, since it is soothing and therapeutic for stress and tension.

Acupressure

There are fourteen acupressure points which should be stimulated in order to reduce Lung stress and strain. (See Illustrations, pages 109 and 111).

Point 1	Crown of head (fontanelle)
Point 2	Posterior fontanelle
Point 3	Anterior fontanelle
Points 4 & 5	Posterior bilateral fontanelle
Points 6 & 7	Anterior bilateral fontanelle
Point 8	7th cervical vertebra (main Air stress point)
Point 9	5th dorsal vertebra (main Air psychological stress point)

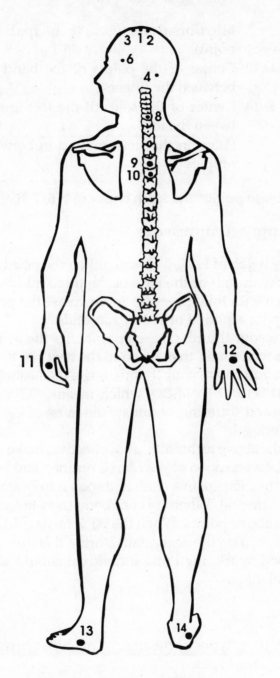

Acupressure Points

Point 10   6th dorsal vertebra (principal anxiety
                  point)
Points 11 & 12   Center of the palms of the hand and in
                  between the fingers
Points 13 & 14   Center of the soles of the feet and in be-
                  tween the toes
Point 15   Point on the sternum and in between the
                  nipples

Out of these points, the main ones are 1, 6, 7, 8, 9, 10 & 15.

How to Apply Acupressure

1. Apply a dab of heated sesame oil on the points.
2. Use the thumb or the base of the three middle fingers. Begin with mild pressure and increase the pressure to deep for a period of 15 to 20 seconds.
3. Rotate your thumb on each point after the acupressure for seven times, then go on to the next point.
4. When you rotate your thumb, recite the healing mantra NAD SOD DHON SOD, which means: "Eliminate the pain and suffering, eliminate the cause of the pain and suffering."

In case the above technique is not effective, make a mixture comprised of a teaspoon of powdered nutmeg and another of barley. Put the mixture in a cloth and soak it in heated melted butter or sesame oil. When it is hot enough to use, apply the pack on the above points. When the pack turns cold, reheat it and then apply it on the next point. During this treatment and the other bodywork, the Lung individual should always be warm in a blanket.

Meditation

The following types of meditative practice are not recommended for Lung types:

• meditation requiring intense concentration

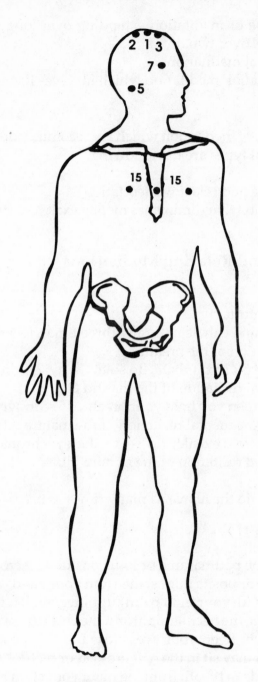

Acupressure Points

- any type of meditation extending over long periods of time, i.e. over two hours
- analytical meditation
- visualization meditation which involves focusing on the heart

The types of meditation which are recommended for Lung constitutional types are the following:

- soothing and relaxing meditation
- meditation that diminishes mental excitation and distraction

Soothing and Relaxing Meditations
Meditation I

1. Sit comfortably.
2. Inhale and exhale naturally three times, focusing on the sensation of the breathing.
3. When you next inhale, do so to the synchronicity of the mental recitation of the mantra OM.
4. Next, when you hold your breath, do so in synchronicity with the mental recitation of the mantra AH.
5. When you exhale, do so to the synchronicity of the mental recitation of the mantra HUNG.

You may do the above as many times as necessary.

Meditation II

1. Sit in the padmasama or lotus position by crossing your legs over the opposite thighs, then join your hands at the level of the navel with your right palm cupping your left palm. Hold the body erect, the neck straight and the chest thrown forward. Do not slouch. Keep your eyes closed. If this position is too difficult, you may sit in the half-crossed or half-lotus position.

2. Take a deep breath from the pit of your stomach through both nostrils as you heave your elbows and shoulders in and upward to a rhythmic count of 5.

3. Without pausing, close your right nostril with your right middle finger and exhale from the left nostril in one long, deep and smooth breath to a rhythmic count of 5.

4. Without pausing, close your left nostril, this time with your left middle finger, and exhale from your right nostril in one long, deep and smooth breath, again to a rhythmic count of 5. REPEAT THE WHOLE EXERCISE THREE TIMES.

5. Without pausing, inhale deeply from both nostrils to a rhythmic count of 5 and then exhale from both nostrils to a rhythmic count of 5.

6. Now, as you begin to inhale gently, lean forward to touch your forehead to the floor to the rhythmic count of 5. Then, as you begin to exhale, gently bring yourself upright, again to the rhythmic count of 5.

REPEAT THE WHOLE EXERCISE THREE TIMES.

Meditation III

1. Sit comfortably and focus on your breath.

2. Imagine an object several feet in front of you.

3. Imagine that the object is blue and emanates a healing ray of light which you absorb.

4. Let your mind focus gently on the healing and relaxing aspect of the object. Avoid any judgmental thoughts, and if distractions occur do not try to fight them, but gently come back to the object of focus.

FIRE (TRIPA) CONSTITUTIONAL TYPES

ENVIRONMENTAL AND BEHAVIORAL CHANGES

- Avoid activities of intense mental and physical stress and strain, especially during the afternoon between Noon and 8 P.M.
- Avoid sleeping during the daytime.
- Avoid excessive exercise.
- Exercise should be for relaxation rather than for competition.
- Avoid excessive and regular exposure to direct sunlight or heat.

- Enjoy the cooling breeze and the ocean.
- Enjoy cooling baths and use cooling oils such as sunflower and sandalwood for massage.

BODYWORK

Deep tissue work or full-body massage with heavy oil should be avoided. Rather, massage should be focused on the specific area of the complaint. Cooling oils such as sandalwood, jasmine or safflower should be used.

Instead of massage, one may spray strong jets of cooling herbal water on tense and tired parts of the body.

Another way to soothe and relax sore and tired muscles for Fire types is through sweating, induced by wrapping the body in a warm blanket.

MEDITATION

Generally, meditations which are goal-oriented — such as those which have proven helpful in relieving stress or medical conditions like high blood pressure — are the kinds which Tripa constitutional types will respond to. Other kinds of meditations — especially those which have an abstract or idealistic content — will not appeal to the Tripa type.

The following types of meditation are recommended:

- clinically proven meditation techniques (including biofeedback) which help reduce stress or medical conditions
- meditations on love and patience

Clinically Proven Meditation Techniques

Meditation I

1. Sit comfortably, back upright.
2. Breathe naturally and smoothly three times.
3. When you are relaxed, inhale and simultaneously contract or tense the heels of your feet in synchronicity with your breathing. As you exhale, relax the heels, again in synchronicity with your breathing.

4. Repeat the same process with the contraction and relaxation of your calves, then the thigh muscles, the stomach, the arms and shoulders and finally the neck.

5. Breathe normally three times.

REPEAT THE WHOLE EXERCISE THREE TIMES.

The above exercise is known as Relaxation Response, and has been used clinically by Dr. Herbert Benson of the Harvard Medical School and found helpful in relieving anxiety, tension, insomnia and other stress-related conditions.

Meditation II (Meditation on Love)

1. Sit comfortably and visualize people you dislike in front of you, people you love dearly behind you, and those whom you do not know on your right and left.

2. Wish sincerely that all of them — especially those you dislike — may attain happiness and bliss. Next, imagine that they have actually attained happiness and bliss. Stay with that image.

3. Observe how long your mind can accept the image of all the people you dislike obtaining happiness through your wish that they may do so.

4. Next, visualize the reality of the condition of all the people surrounding you. All of them are in some way caught up in their suffering and pain. Recognize their pain and suffering visually in your mind.

5. Now, generate a fervent wish to see them attain liberation from that pain and suffering by mentally chanting these words: "May my enemies and those that I do not like and need not like, those that I do not know and care for, and those I deeply care for and love with all my heart, all equally and without any differentiation attain happiness and freedom from pain."

WATER (BAGAN) CONSTITUTIONAL TYPES

ENVIRONMENTAL AND BEHAVIORAL CHANGES

- Avoid sleeping more than seven to eight hours a night, and definitely avoid sleeping during any part of the day.

- Avoid strenuous and stressful activities during the early mornings or late evenings.
- Engage in strenuous, movement-oriented exercises on a regular basis.
- Avoid exposure to damp, wet ground or weather. Get as much sunlight and heat as possible.
- Avoid too much exposure to water or cooling breezes.
- Seek all types of sensory stimulation; avoid using a single sensory organ all the time, as in watching television durng your daily relaxation period.

BODYWORK

Deep tissue work with the use of minimal or no oils is recommended. Full body massage is not recommended. However, cleansing the body with chickpea flour after a massage is highly recommended for Bagan types.

MEDITATION

In general, the type of meditation recommended for Water types is active and stimulating rather than sedating, withdrawing and relaxing. This is because the Water person is already predisposed to withdrawal and dullness, which meditation may tend to increase. As a result, stimulating, active, and externally focused meditations are recommended.

Meditation I

1. Sit comfortably and breathe naturally three times.

2. When you complete a respiratory cycle, mentally count it as 1 and the next one as 2. Count up to 10.

3. After the tenth cycle, count the next cycle as 9 and go backwards to 1.

REPEAT THE EXERCISE THREE TIMES.

Meditation II

1. Sit comfortably and visualize your mind as a bright ball of pure light, the size of a marble. Imagine that the ball is localized in your heart.

2. Next, imagine that when you loudly recite the mantra PHAT, the ball of light which is your mind shoots straight up your body and out the crown of your head, into space.
REPEAT THIS EXERCISE THREE OR MORE TIMES.

Behavior and Spiritual Practice

Spiritual behavior is defined by Buddhists *as engaging in the path of wisdom and compassion in order to obtain characteristics which will allow us to work efficiently for the benefit of others and, in the process, attain our own liberation.* Merely obtaining the pleasure and comforts of the five senses is temporary and does not involve the true purpose of human life. The following are some of the basic steps in spiritual practice and behavior.

- Identify your purpose and your need for a spiritual practice.
- Identify your motivation for seeking a spiritual practice.
- Identify your present values and belief system.
- Seek an authentic source for information about a spiritual path. It might be worth your while to spend time in finding an appropriate teacher, i.e. a teacher who lives by what he or she preaches, uses authentic resources and literature in teaching, and has a genuine, grounded group of practitioners.
- Study, listen and then contemplate on what you have been taught. Spend at least 30 minutes a day in contemplation.
- Spend one weekend per month on retreat.
- Plan your spiritual practice in connection with your other priorities in life and in consultation with your spiritual guide.
- From time to time, evaluate your spiritual practice and examine how it has affected your behavior over the last six months.
- Keep a diary of major spiritual events, teachings you have received, and retreats you have undertaken.

For those who seek seriously to enhance the maintenance of their physical health through spiritual practice, we shall devote the next two chapters to a specific program of basic spiritual work.

7
TIBETAN PANCHA KARMA:
Mind-body Integration Treatment

INTRODUCTION

Tibetan pancha karma treatment originated in Ayurveda, the Hindu "science of life;" however, the Tibetans have modified pancha karma in order to suit local needs and environmental differences. Though pancha karma has been virtually non-existent in Tibet for several centuries, the Institute of Tibetan Buddhist Wellness and Counseling is beginning to revive its practice.

In Tibetan, pancha karma is called Las Nga, meaning "the five actions," the five detoxifying, rejuvenating and therapeutic techniques. Pancha karma is used for both therapeutic and preventative purposes. Therapeutically, it is highly recommended for a variety of disorders ranging from psychological problems such as anxiety and depression to physical complaints such as arthritis, gastro-intestinal problems, neuromuscular disorders, etc. We will cover the use and benefits of pancha karma for health maintenance and psycho-physical integration.

The five major cleansing, regenerative, and therapeutic techniques are enemas, purgatives, emetics (vomiting), nasal stimulation, and blood detoxification. In addition, there are secondary forms of pancha karma such as dripping oil on parts of the body, herbal packs, etc.

Any form of pancha karma treatment consists of two parts: preliminary treatment and actual treatment.

PRELIMINARY TREATMENT

OIL THERAPHY

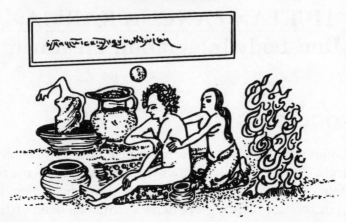

Preliminary treatment is designed to prepare the client for the actual pancha karma and itself involves two forms of treatment. The first part consists of oleation and massage, which involves selecting the appropriate oil, typically an herbal medicated oil, and applying it to the client's body for stimulation and massage. This is not only to relax the client, his muscles, and his body, but also to stimulate and excite toxins within the superficial parts of the body such as the muscles and skin, and to encourage the internal toxins to collect in the gastro-intestinal region for elimination.

HERBAL STEAMING AND BATH

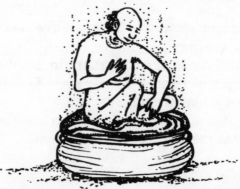

Following oleation and massage is herbal steaming in a steam cabinet for an interval between fifteen and thirty minutes. Various combinations of herbs are used, depending on the constitutional typology of the client, but the most popular is known as the five herbal nectars, which consists of five Himalayan herbs. The purpose of the herbal steaming is to further relax the muscles and, primarily, to eliminate external toxins from the muscles and skin through the process of sweating and steaming. This preliminary combined treatment, in addition to the effects stated above, also helps to improve complexion, reduce weight, improve clarity, and cleanse the skin.

THE FIVE TREATMENTS OF PANCHA KARMA

The combinations of pancha karma treatment will vary for each client depending upon constitutional typology and the nature of the complaint. However, the general recommendation for pancha karma is as follows:

Enemas	For Lung complaints or constitutions
Purgatives	For Tripa complaints or constitutions
Emetics	For Bagan complaints or constitutions
Nasal stimulation	For allergies, headaches, and sinus problems
Blood Detoxification	For yeast infections, blood-related allergies, and bloodtoxicity

Traditionally, the duration of pancha karma treatment varies depending on whether it is used for medical or for preventative, rejuvenating purposes. When it is used for medical purposes the treatment is regular and prolonged, involving many sessions, while for rejuvenating and preventative purposes the duration of the treatment is confined to fewer sessions based on seasonal changes.

To determine the type of pancha karma to use, an initial history and evaluation is absolutely necessary. The evaluation involves doing a physical, checking urine and pulse, and questioning, as well as taking a history of past medical information.

ACTUAL PANCH KARMA

EMESIS

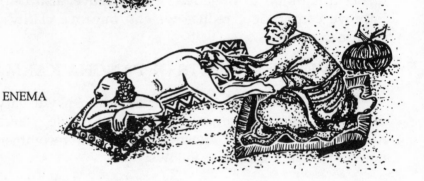

ENEMA

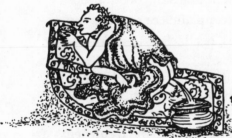

PURGATIVES

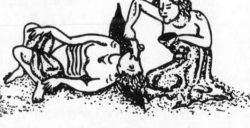

NASAL THERAPHY

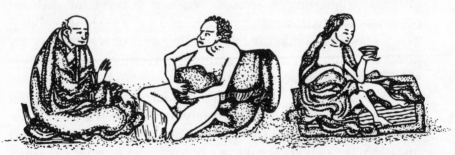

FOMETATION

CHANNEL PURIFICATION

USES OF ENEMAS, PURGATIVES AND EMETICS

Enemas:	Used Therapeutically when Lung Disorders Manifest
These Include:	Constipation, Distension, Lower Back Pain, Sciatica, Arthritis, Nervousness, Tension, Headaches, Emaciation and Muscular Distrophy
Used Prophylactically for Air Types, Primarily in Summer	
Purgatives:	Used Therapeutically when Tripa Disorders Manifest
These Include:	Chronic Fever, Worms, Jaundice and Skin Diseases
Used Prophylactically for Fire Types, Primarily in Late Summer and Early Autumn	
Emetics:	Used Therapeutically When Bagan Disorders Manifest
These Include:	Coughs, Colds, Nausea, Loss of Appetite, Respiratory Illnesses, Chronic Sinus Problems and Lymphatic Obstructions
Used Prophylactically for Water Types, Primarily Beginning in Spring	

Based on the evaluation, the combination of pancha karma treatments is determined. The program may also include secondary pancha karma treatment such as oil dripping, herbal packs, etc., in addition to enemas, purgatives, emetics, nasal stimulation or blood detoxification.

Oil dripping treatment (shiridara) is an adjunct to pancha karma designed to facilitate a calm, blissful state of consciousness in which to carry out healing through visualization. Heated sesame oil is normally used. The client lies on a massage table and the oil drips on the subtle point between and above the eyebrows (the "third eye"). For the first five minutes the oil drips, and for the next ten minutes the oil flows on the point. During the dripping and flowing of the oil, the client is required to withdraw his mental functions to the sensation of the oil dripping, and in this way to enter into a calm and relaxed state of mind. The client is then required to focus on the sensation and dripping of the oil, which stimulates a sense of intense bliss. When a calm and blissful state is experienced, the client is encouraged to examine any image he experiences.

Following the oil dripping, the nasal and facial treatment is administered. This involves an application of oil on the face, followed by a facial massage and then a hot pack fomentation. To cool the eyes and clean the skin, cucumber slices are kept on the eyes during the application of the heated packs. Once the facial massage and pack is over, nasal stimulation treatment follows. Depending on the complaint and constitutional typology of the client, different herbal drips are used. The most common is ginger and brown sugar liquid dripped into the nostrils. This particular nasal medication helps to clear the sinuses, improve memory, generate energy in the brain, improve circulation and tone neuro-muscular functioning in the body.

In Air (Lung) conditions and typologies, a nutritional herbal milk massage follows, to tone, strengthen, and nourish the skin and muscles. Following this treatment, it is recommended that the client perform cleansing by means of enemas, purgatives, or emetics at home. For clients who have blood toxic conditions, herbal blood cleansers are recommended.

In addition to the above, nutritional guidelines are used to recommend a diet for the period of pancha karma treatment as well as a long-term diet plan. Whenever necessary, nutritional herbs are recommended to enhance the vitality and harmony of the energy systems in the body.

PANCHA KARMA TREATMENTS FOR THE THREE TYPOLOGIES

	Air (Lung)	Fire (Tripa)	Water (Bagan)
1	Whole Body Massage with Sesame Oil	Light Massage or No Massage without Jasmine Oil or Sandalwood Oil	Deep Tissue Massage with oil
2	Herbal Steaming	Herbal Steaming	Herbal Steaming
3	Shiridara	Nasaya	Nasaya
4	Counseling	Shirada	Shirada Counseling
5	Nasaya	Purgatives	Hot Packs
6	Nurturing Massage		Emetics
7	Enemas		

8
HERBAL
THERAPEUTICS

INTRODUCTION

While Tibetan pharmacology is unique, it has incorporated much of the Ayurvedic herbal system as well as parts of the Chinese in order to create a complete and integrated system of herbs. Prior to the advent of the famous Buddhist teacher Nagarjuna in India, Ayurveda was primarily an herbal system of healing. Nagarjuna introduced the art of alchemy, and soon the use of gems, precious metals, and minerals as therapeutic substances became a fascinating component of Ayurveda. When Ayurveda came to Tibet, the Tibetans also incorporated the use of gems, precious metals, animal parts and minerals along with the herbs, and compounded more than several thousand healing formulations. However, herbology remains an entity in itself, and the use of pure herbs as therapeutic agents still prevails. Tibetan pharmacological literature deals extensively with the potentials of herbs, both individually and in combination. Here we will deal with herbs that can be commonly used by the individual as self-healing agents at home. The use of herbs as therapeutic agents as described here is for personal home use and not intended as a substitute for medical treatment.

THERAPEUTIC HERBS

Some of the herbs listed here may not be available from regular herb stores, except from Indian herbal stores or from the Institute of Tibetan Buddhist Wellness and Counseling.

Angelica (Angelica archangelica): The dried root has a pungent, bittersweet taste and a warming, therapeutic effect on the body. It is anti-Air as well as anti-Air-Water, and tends to increase Fire. Angelica root, when taken as a powder or decoction, is helpful for opening the body vessels in general and is an effective diuretic. It increases digestive heat and relieves cold and hay fever.

Aniseed has a pungent taste and a warming, therapeutic effect on the body. It is a useful digestive aid, relieving flatulence and distension. Aniseed is anti-Air and is more neutral in its effect on the other two Nepas in the body. It may be taken as a powder or decoction.

Asafoetida: The resin or powder of asafoetida has a pungent, strong odor and taste and a warming effect. It is excellent for flatulence, a natural laxative, anti-spasmodic, and a digestive aid. It also promotes circulation. It is anti-Air and anti-Water but tends to increase Fire. It may be taken in very small quantities as a decoction or in powder form. A pinch of asafoetida cooked with lentils helps digestion and relieves gas.

Ashwagandha (Withania somnifera): The root of ashwagandha is bittersweet in taste and has a slightly warming effect on the body. Taken as a powder or decoction, it is a tonic, rejuvenative, aphrodisiac, sedative and diuretic. It increases kidney heat and is anti-Water.

Asparagus racemosis root has a sweet, bitter taste and cooling effect, and is good for bronchitis, chronic lung disorders, constipation, diabetes, and lymphatic congestion and swelling. It also serves as a tonic, rejuvenative, and aphrodisiac. It may be taken as a powder or decoction.

Black pepper (Piper Nigrum) is a pungent stimulant which increases digestive heat. A pinch or more may be sprinkled in meals. It is anti-Air and anti-Water but increases Fire.

Cardamom (Elettaria cardamomum — green seeds) has a bitter, pungent taste and a warming effect. Taken as an infusion or powder or even with meals, cardamom serves as a stimulant and carminative, and is good for poor circulation, abdominal cramps, gas, indigestion and malabsorption. It is a kidney stimulant. It is anti-Water and anti-Air but increases Fire.

Cinnamon: The bark, taken in powder or as an infusion, has a pungent, sweet taste and a warming effect on the body. It increases body heat and is good for diarrhea, gas, cold stomach, cough, asthma, toothache, and nerve pain.

Coriander, taken as an infusion or powder, is simply cooked with vegetables and is a stimulant, carminative, alterative, and digestive aid. It has a sweet, pungent taste and neutral effect on the body.

Clove seeds, taken in powder form in tea or cooked in food, have a bitter, pungent taste and a warming effect on the body. They are a digestive aid. They relive pain and also alleviate coughs, congestion, colds and sinus problems. Clove is anti-Water and anti-Air but may increase Fire slightly.

Cumin seeds, taken in powdered form in food or as a pinch in milk, help to relieve abdominal pain and cramps, and increase body heat because of their bitter and pungent taste.

Cucumber seeds have a bitter taste and a cooling effect on the body. They help to eliminate heat disorders and inflammation in the stomach and intestine and are also good for hemorrhoids. They are anti-Fire but increase Air and Water.

Dandelion root is bittersweet in taste and has a cooling effect on the body. It may be taken in the form of an infusion, decoction, or powder for liver dysfunction, jaundice, gall stones and congested lymph nodes. Dandelion increases Water and Air.

Eaglewood (Aquilaria agollocha) bark powder is bitter and pungent in taste and has a slightly warming and heavy effect on the body. Taken as a decoction, it is an excellent relaxant, sedative and nervine tonic.

Ephedra root is pungent, bitter, and astringent in taste and has a warming effect on the body. Taken in the form of a decoction, it helps aches, pains, colds and chills, and induces sweating.

Fennel (Foeniculum vulgare) seeds may be taken as an infusion or in powdered form. Their bitter, pungent, and warming effect is an excellent digestive aid. They increase stomach and spleen heat and help stomach pain and cramps.

Garlic (Allum staivum) has a pungent taste and a warming effect. Taken in food or powdered form, it is recommended for chills, for elimination of toxicity and gas, and for general Air conditions. Garlic is generally anti-Air and anti-Water and may increase Fire slightly.

Ginger has a pungent, astringent taste and a warming effect on the body. Taken as an infusion or with food, it helps to dilute blood, raise digestive heat and heat of the spleen, reduce pain and gas as well as congestion and coughs, and clear the sinuses.

Gotu Kola (Hyedrocotyle asistica): The leaf of the Gotu Kola is taken in powdered form to cleanse mucus and sinuses and to stimulate the brain tissues and memory.

Hibiscus has a sweet taste and cooling effect, and is recommended for diarrhea, skin eruptions and rashes, yeast infection, difficult or painful menstruation, and cystitis. It may be taken as an infusion or powder. Hibiscus is anti-Fire and tends to increase Water and Air.

Raisins (black) may be taken directly or cooked with rice, etc., to help with colds, flu, sore throat or chronic lung disorders. They have a sweet taste and a cooling effect on the body.

Turmeric taken in powdered form with food has a bitter and cooling effect and helps to eliminate toxins, heal wounds when applied to them, reduce infection and inflammation, and heal hemorrhoids. Turmeric may also be taken in a decoction.

Safflower seeds have a sweet and cooling effect. They help stop bleeding, improve anemic conditions, and detoxify the liver.

Saffron is much cooler and more potent than safflower. It has the same therapeutic effects as safflower and is normally cooked with rice.

Sesame seeds have a pungent and sharp taste and a warming effect on the body. Taken with food, they increase digestive heat and generally strengthen the body.

Solomon's seal (Polygonatum cirrhifolium) root is sweet and neutral.

Stinging nettle leaves have a pungent, bitter taste and heating quality. They are excellent as a soup for Air disorders such as insomnia and stress. They are also effective as a diuretic when taken with tea.

General Air (Lung) Formulations

Aquilaria 35 is recommended for flu, chills, joint pain, insomnia, upper back pain and tension, anxiety and hyperventilation.

Aquilaria 18 is recommended for depression, anxiety, pain in the chest, and mental disorientation.

Vimalamitra is recommended for hysteria, feelings of emptiness, disassociation, anxiety and panic attacks.

General Fire (Tripa) Formulations

Tikta 25 (Felwort 25) is recommended for both cold and hot Tripa disorders with symptoms as follows: headache, bitter taste in the mouth, lethargy, nausea, indigestion. Take 1 pill with water before lunch.

Tikta 25 is composed of Swertia chirata, Swertia petiolata, Phlogacanthus pubinervius, Herpetospermum caudgerum, Holarrhena antidysenterica, Vitis vinifera, Gentiana tibertica, Aconitum herterophyllum, Myristica fragrans, Terminalia chebula, Saussurea lappa, Bambusa textilis, mineral pitch, Veronica ciliata, Punica granatum, Carthamus tinctorius, Elettaria cardamomum, Piper longum, bear's bile, Eugenia caryophyllata, Acacia catechu, Datura sp., Arenaria glanduligera, lac, and Sabina recurva.

Serdog 11 (Golden color 11) is recommended for Tripa conditions with symptoms such as pain in the stomach, intestine, liver and gall baldder; nausea and headache; gall stones; and halitosis or bitter taste in the mouth. Take 1 pill before lunch.

Serdog 11 is prepared from Terminalia chebula, black camphor, Aconitum heterophyllum, Embvelia ribes, musk, Aconitum spicatum, Hypercoum leptocarpum, mineral pitch, Punica granatum, Herpetospermum caudgerum, and Rosa sericea.

General Bagan Formulations

Sedru 5 (Pomegranate 5) is recommended to increase stomach heat, as a digestive and carminative, and to relieve pain in the kidneys and hips due to lack of stomach heat. Take 1 pill before breakfast.

Sedru 5 is composed of Punica granatum, Cinnamomum zeylanicum, Piper longum, Elettaria cardamomum, and Hedychium spicatum.

Ruta 6 (Saussurea 6) is a generic formula for gastritis, colic, eructation, inflammation of the stomach, emesis and nausea, and flatulence. Take 1 pill with warm water before breakfast.

Ruta 6 is composed of Saussurea lappa, Embblica officinalis, Punica granatum, Veronica ciliata, Elettaria cardamomum, and Piper longum.

QUALITIES OF HERBS AND HERBAL FORMULAS

HERB	NATURE • TASTE	THERAPY • ACTION	ENERGETIC EFFECT	FOODS • PREPARATION	COMPLIMENTARY HERB
Angelica Angelica archangelica Dried roots	Warming Sweet · Bitter · Hot	Rejuvenates blood. Opens BV's & other bodily channels. Good for fluid retention. Diuretic, raises heat.	Air Water Air	Cook the root in water until soft, can be eaten as a vegetable or made into a soup COOKED	Cumin
Aniseed/Anise Seed	Warming Hot · Pungent	Digestive aid. Relieves flatulence. Lowers body heat.	Air	Meats, eggs, cheese, vegetables stewed fruits SAUTEED · SPRINKLED INTO A DISH AS IT'S COOKING	Coriander · Cumin Ginger
Asfoetida Resin, Powder	Warming Hot · Pungent	Digestive aid. Relieves flatulence. Raises body heat.	Air Water	Beans, grains, meats, vegetables No dairy or eggs SAUTEED OR SPRINKLED	Cumin · Coriander Tumeric · Jaggery
Ashwaganda / Withania sonnifera · Dried root	Neutral Sweet · Bitter	Diuretic, rejuvanative. Raises kidney heat.	Water	Cook the dried root as a separate dish	Cardamom · Cumin Coriander · Ginger
Barberry Berberis vulgaris Bark-dried & powdered	Cooling Bitter	Eliminates inflammation & diarrhea.	Fire	Cooked into oily, greasy foods such as meat	Jaggery or honey may be added to kill bitterness
Black Pepper Piper nigrum	Heating Hot · Pungent	Stimulant. Raises digestive heat	Water	Vegetables, meats SAUTEED OR SPRINKLED	Cumin · Coriander Turmeric
Cayenne Pepper/Capsicum frutescens · Chili	Heating Hot · Pungent	Raises digestive heat. Eliminates growth & tumors, micro-organisms, hemorrhoids. Fluid retention.	Water Air-occais	Soups, Stews, vegetables SPRINKLED	Cumin · Coriander Turmeric
Cardamom Eletaria cardamomum (green) · Seed	Warming Hot · Bitter	Raises body heat & digestive heat. Good for the immune system.	Water Air	Tea, milk, desserts, rice, root vegetables, meatballs, meat. COOKED PODS FOR MILD USE (PILAFS) GROUND FOR AROMATIC USE IN PUDDINGS	Cinnamon · Ginger Cumin Coriander
Cinnamon/Cinnamomum zeylonica · Bark-powder	Heating Hot · Sweet	Induces body heat. Good for diarrhea, gas, cold stomach, liver.	Air · Water Fire	Desserts, fruit dishes, vegetables, meat, tea SPRINKLED	Cardamom · Clove Fennel · Ginger
Clove Seed, Powder	Heating Hot · Bitter	Digestive aid. Improves body heat. Relieves anxiety, tension.	Water Air	Pilafs, rice, soups, root vegetables, meat, tea COOKED	Coriander · Cumin Ginger · Nutmeg
Coriander/Coriandrum Sativum · Seed	Neutral Hot · Sweet · Salty	Raises digestion. Improves appetite. Gastritis.	Air/Fire	Salads, meat, vegetables, curries SAUTEED, SPRINKLED	Cumin · Fennel · Garlic Ginger · Turmeric
Cucumber Seeds	Cooling Bitter	Eliminates heating disorder, inflammation. Especially in stomach & intestines. Good for piles, hemorrhoids.	Fire	Tea	
Cumin Seed, Powder	Warming Hot · Pungent Bitter	Raises body heat. Good for digestion, stomach.	Air Water	Soups, meats, vegetables SAUTEED	Fennel · Garlic Ginger · Turmeric Coriander

HERB	NATURE • TASTE	THERAPY • ACTION	EFFECT	FOODS • PREPARATION	HERB
Dandelion/Tarraxacum officinale · Root	Cooling Bitter · Sweet	Fever. Stomach, liver, joints (inflammation).	Fire	Tea	
Eaglewood (aqualaria) Root, Branches, Powder	Neutral Bitter · Hot	Anxiety. Nerve relaxant	Fire Heat	Grains, meats, tea, vegetables SAUTÉED	Clove · Cumin · Garlic Coriander · Ginger
Ephedra Root	Warming Hot · Bitter · Astringent	Aches, pains. Induces sweating. Colds, chills, excessive sweating.	Fire	Tea or dried root cooked in honey/water. May be eaten alone as a snack	
Fennel/Foeniculum vulgare · Seed, Powder	Warming Bitter · Hot	Digestive aid. Raises stomach & spleen heat. Eliminates pain.	Water Air	Desserts, pastries, tea, okra, vegetables/stir fry, soups, meat · SPRINKLED, COOKED	Asafoetida · Coriander Cuimin · Ginger
Fenugreek/Trigonella foenumgraecum · Seed	Neutral · Warming · Bitter Pungent · Sweet · (hot)		Water Air	Tea or roasted & used in pickling or lightly in vegetarian dishes	
Garlic/Allium sativum Pod (bulb)	Heating Pungent (hot)	Chill, fevers. Eliminates micro-organisms & toxicity. Skin disorders & rashes. Stimulant especially heart.	Water/Air Heat Water Air	Butter, cheese, rice, meat, vegetables, or alone with honey · COOKED, SAUTÉED, SPRINKLED	Cumin · Coriander Ginger · Turmeric
Gentian/Seniana lutea Root	Cooling Bitter	General heat conditions as hepatitis, jaundice. Lowers liver, gallbladder heat.	Fire	Tea	Saffron Sugar/Honey
Ginger/Zingiberis officinalis · Root, dried, fresh	Warming Hot · Pungent · Astringent	Dilutes blood. Raises digestive body heat, also spleen heat. Lowers cold conditions. Removes pain, gas.	Water Air	Desserts, Grains, rice, relishes, meats, vegetables, tea · SAUTÉED OR SPRINKLED, JUICE	Cumin · Coriander Turmeric · Onion
Gotu kola/Hyedrocotyle asiatica · Leaf	Cooling Bitter	Diarrhea. Liver, lung infections. Skin eruptions, rashes.	Fire	Tea	Honey
Guggul/Indian Bedellium Resin	Cooling Bitter	Eliminates infections and inflammation. Heals sores & wounds.	Fire	Tea	Honey
Hibiscus · Flowers picked in Autumn	Cooling Sweet, Smooth	Diarrhea, loose stool. Skin Eruptions & rashes. Stops vaginal discharge, yeast infection.	Fire	Tea BOILED	
Jaggery Rock Powdered or Melted	Warming Sweet Nourishing	Fatigue, muscle tension. Dizziness, stress. Raises body heat. Rejuvenates body strength.	Air	Desserts, grains, rice, vegetables, meat, tea	Ginger Aqualaria
Licorice Glycyrrhiza glabra Powdered Roots	Neutral Sweet	Cough & respiratory problems. Eliminates fever. Eliminates vomiting and sore throats.	Water Fire	Beverages, desserts, tea BOILED	Ginger Cinnamon
Long Pepper/Pippali Piper longum	Heating Hot · Sweet	Raises body heat & digestive fire. Lungs, spleen. Respiratory disorders.	Water Air	Grains, vegetables, soups SPRINKLED	Cumin · Coriander Turmeric
Nutmeg Myristica fragrans Seed	Warming Hot Pungent	Anxiety, tension. Palpition, heart pain. Digestion. Insomnia, sedative.	Air	Chutneys, tea, fruit conserves, soups, vegetable, chicken, puddings, yogurt. BOILED, SPRINKLED IN SMALL QUANTITIES (1/2 TEASPOON)	

HERB	NATURE • TASTE	THERAPY • ACTION	ENERGETIC EFFECT	FOODS • PREPARATION	COMPLIMENTARY HERB
Onions Allium cepa	Warming Sweet, Hot	Raises appetite, digestion. Dizziness, forgetfulness. Ringing ears. Insomnia.	Water/Air	Eggs, meat, vegetables, soup, stews. SAUTEED, FIRST SPICES IN GHEE, ADD ONION, COOK, ADD WATER, SIMMER AND ADD OTHER MAIN INGREDIENTS	May Be Used With Only Spices
Raisins Black	Cooling Sweet	Colds, flu, sore throats, respiratory asthma. Chronic Air disorders. Eliminates Air inflammation.	Fire Water	Desserts, grains, rice, salads COOKED IN WITH THE INGREDIENTS	
Rhododendron Flowers	Cooling Bitter	Kidney infections. Poisoning. Stops Bleeding. Regulates Menses.	Fire	Tea	
Rose/Rosa macrophylla Pink/Red · Fruit, heart of flower	Neutral Sweet · Sour Bitter	Stops seminal discharge (male/female). Diarrhea.	Fire	Tea	
Rose/Rosa sericea Yellow Whole Plant	Cooling Bitter	Fevers. Induces menstration. Tumors. Ovarian cysts.	Fire	Tea	
Safflower/Carthamus Tinctorius · Seed	Cooling Sweet	Bleeding, Blood, anemic conditions. Detoxification & purification. Liver conditions.	Fire	Rice vegetables SPRINKLED	
Saffron/Crocus sativa Stamen	Cooler Stronger than Safflower		Fire	Puddings, pilaf, almond Halwa	
Sandalwood/Santalum alba White	Cooling Astringent	Fever, inflammation skin, heart, lungs, muscles.	Fire	Tea	
Sandalwood/Santalum alba Red	Cooling Astringent	Blood, heat and wind disorder, purifying, lowers external swelling if applied externally.	Blood	Tea	
Sesame (white & black) Seeds (when toasted makes more digestible)	Heating Pungent · Sharp (penetrating)	Raises body heat body weight and strengthens body.	Air Water	Desserts, soup, meat, vegetables SPRINKLED, COOKED	
Shatavari/Asparagus racemosus · Root	Cooling Sweet · Bitter	Bronchitis. Chronic Air disorders. Constipation, coughing, diabetes, lymph swelling.	Fire Air	Cook the root as a side dish (SIMMERED IN WATER TO SOFTEN)	
Shilagit (mineral Pitch) Exudate (tarry Resin)	Warming Sweet	Cramps, irregular menses, intestinal cramps.	Fire	Tea MUST BE HEATED IN PURE ALCOHOL · 2 TABLESPOONS OF HERB TO 4-5 TABLESPOONS OF ALCOHOL UNTIL ALCOHOL EVAPORATES	
Stinging Nettle Urticadioica	Heating Pungent, Bitter	Raises body heat. Sedative (all Air conditions).	Air	Soups	Cumin · Coriander Pinch Nutmeg

HERB	NATURE • TASTE	THERAPY • ACTION	ENERGETIC EFFECT	FOODS • PREPARATION	COMPLIMENTARY HERB
Solomon's Seal Polygonatum cirrhifolium Root	Neutral, Sweet	Raises body strength, temperature. Diuretic, kidney pain, bloating excess joint fluid. Skin rash & eruptions.	Air	Serve as side dish or with onions in various dishes COOKED, GRATED OR POWDERED UNTIL SOFT	Onions
Triphala or Myrobalin 1) Haritaki/Terminalia chebula Fruit, Powder	Neutral Astringent	Common cold flu, sore throat, chronic flu:ng, kidneys, stops diarrhea, rejuvenating.	Air, Water/Fire	Tea	
2) Bibhitaki/Terminalia belerica Fruit, Powder	Neutral Astringent	Cleansing effect to the whole body, dries excess fluid especially from the lymphatic system.	Water/Fire	Tea	
3) Amalaki/Emblica officinalis Fruit	Cooling Sour	Blood purifier, hot liver condition, hair loss.	Water, Air, Hot Blood	Tea	
Turmeric Curcuma longa Powder	Cooling Bitter	Eliminates toxins. Heals wounds, sores. Eliminates infection & inflammation, piles, hemorrhoids.	Fire Water	Grains, rice, vegetables, meat, lentil stews SAUTEED IN GHEE (ROOTS MAY BE EATEN AS VEGETABLES)	Ginger Cumin Coriander

HERBS AND DISORDERS

Drug	1 smooth	2 heavy	3 warm	4 oily	5 stable	6 cold	7 blunt	8 cool
Disorder	coarse	light	cold	subtle	mobile	oily	sharp	hot
				hard				

Drug	9 soft	10 moist	11 dry	12 pale	13 hot	14 light	15 sharp	16 coarse	17 mobile
Disorder	light	foul odor	purgative	oily	cool	heavy	blunt	smooth	stable
		moist						sticky	

In order to treat the disorders of Air (Lung), Fire (Tripa) and Water (Badgen) with herbs and diet, the seventeen therapeutic qualities of drugs (herbs and diet) are applied to work against the 20 pathological states of the three disorders (6 pathological conditions for Air, 7 for Fire and 7 for Water). If a skin disorder is primarily rough and coarse then herbs and diet that have smooth, soft qualities are used.

9
BEGINNING
A SPIRITUAL PRACTICE

We have lost touch with a deep part of ourselves, including our religious symbolism and ritual, so that often we can no longer use these tools as part of a spiritual path. However, through a process of spiritual work which we shall define here, we can rediscover how to reconnect. To do so does not require a particular dogmatic belief system, but a willingness to look within.

Although this work is similar to other systems, it does have some unique features because it is Buddhist. In addition, it differs from many other Buddhist systems in its use of Tantric methods involving the use of imagination and emotion to promote spiritual growth. Many of its techniques are similar to the techniques of Jungian psychology. These chapters will explain the essence of Tibetan spiritual practice outside of its cultural and religious context.

One important value not shared by some traditions is the emphasis which Tibetan Buddhism places on bringing our spirituality back into the world. As a form of Mahayana Buddhism it maintains that if our spiritual practice neglects to bridge the gap between our private spiritual experiences and our lives, we will end up thnking that these are two different things. Then we are only spiritual in church on Sunday, or when we meditate. The rest of the time we are not. And if our spiritual practice becomes split off from our everyday lives, we cannot nurture it — or our world.

We believe that what makes a spiritual tradition worthwhile are the universal themes it contains and which can inspire us deeply. Therefore, in the face of great pain and suffering we may turn to such a tradition and find that not only can it acknowledge and host our suffering and pain, it can also connect us to the deeper meaning of such experiences. To merely acknowledge suffering is not enough. Our traditions must help us find a meaning in our suffering. Because Tibetan Buddhism places a high value on the integration of the spiritual and the mundane, maintaining that only when we integrate the two can our spiritual lives sustain us through crisis, it contains many techniques to help us find such meanings.

The path we follow on our quest for spirituality, growth, and transformation is divided into two stages, one of which is preliminary and the other of which is the main portion; each stage consists of multiple steps which we can express as questions. Throughout the process we must ask ourselves:

What does a spiritual practice mean to me?

What are some of the things I might be doing that are frustrating my process?

How would I like to change what I am doing now?

How would I like to see myself next month in my spiritual path?

How would I like to see my changes take place?

DEFINING SPIRITUALITY

Spirituality tends to mean something different to each of us. Before we can begin, we must define what we mean by it here. In addition, we must discover what it means to each of us personally, and honor that meaning in our spiritual work.

The East actually has no word meaning "spiritual." The closest is *dharum*, which means "that which holds to its true nature." This word is usually translated as religion. Some interpret it as "that which keeps us from suffering and pain" or "that which protects us." So it is similar to the word refuge. But its real meaning is "that which holds to its true nature." When we hold to our true nature, then we are spiritual in the Buddhist sense. Holding to our true nature means to actualize the Inner Self.

What is the Inner Self? Most of us think of it as something unconscious, pure, immaculate and inacessible. Once in a while we get a glimpse of it in the form of a numinous experience or profound insight. To gain full access to it, we must complete all twelve steps of the path outlined below. Since we have not done so yet, we must use symbols when we talk about the Self, though it is not any of our symbols. It isn't a refuge, a teacher, God, love, or compassion. These are positive qualities which most of us want to identify as the Inner Self. However, when we get a sense of the Self through meditation, we will realize that it is more than just these positive qualities.

According to Tibetan Buddhism, spiritual practice does not imply that you live by any particular code of ethics and morality in the world; rather, it stresses numerous ways in which you need to tap into your inner world as a way of being more naturally in the outer world. In other words, knowing your true self, its potential and inner dynamics is an integral part of the spiritual path. When you can travel into the inner world of your psyche and acknowledge its presence and powers, you can accept the changing, uncertain, impermanent qualities of the outer world with more courage. Spiritual health involves finding the natural rhythm among your inner parts so that they can synchronize with your emotional, physical and outer world.

Spiritual health involves finding the inner center of your being and letting it guide your ego towards wholeness and growth. When the ego is alienated from the inner center or Self, meaning and purpose in life exist only in terms of the emotional, physical and mundane. When outer events no longer give you the same stimulation, the ego suffers and is displaced, since this is the only way in which the ego is capable of defining happiness. When the inner Self is active and helps the ego to maneuver in the world, then your inner world will become a rich imaginal source of meaning and exploration into untouched, undiscovered parts of yourself during those times and situations when the outer world fails you.

Spiritual health gives us a sense of constancy that is crucial to our physical and psychological health. The world has become so complex, so changing and fluid that it is virtually impossible to keep up with the changes that are taking place. Unless we have an inner constancy we may easily begin to feel psychically displaced.

MINDFULNESS

Before we embark on the path we must develop the basic skills we will need. They are the skills common to most spiritual traditions.

The most basic prerequisite is mindfulness, in order to develop a quiet, focused state of mind which permits us to be mindful or aware of immediate experience. It is also called "calm abiding", because our minds are calm but focused and abiding on some object. Once we can maintain our focus on the object for some time, we gradually reduce the effort required to maintain focus while still maintaining awareness. The less effort needed to maintain the focus, the greater is our calm abiding skill. Tension reduction is crucial because tension makes our practice rigid and unhealthy. Our goal is pliancy: a relaxed but focused state. This produces a resiliency which allows us to host analytical or insight meditation, the next step. Developing mindfulness and pliancy of mind will change our daily lives by increasing our awareness of what we experience. Then we will realize we are angry before we have acted out and begun to feel guilty. Pliancy helps us tolerate unpleasant emotional states like anger and fear. Then, instead of being driven by our anger, we can decide what to do about it.

Insight Meditation

Insight meditation is a form of analytical self-analysis which we can use in order to obtain insight into our actions and uncover the blocks to our spiritual growth. It can help us figure out how we perceive other people, our true attitudes regarding a specific issue, or what our resistances are. However, it can only give us intellectual answers to these questions — it will not necessarily free us from the problem. In order to find freedom, we must usually move on to the third type of meditation, the imaginal or Tantric.

Imaginal Work

Imaginal work or Tantric meditation uses the imagination to further explore what we have learned from our insight work. We do this by fantasizing a story which we can use to produce transformation. This is possible because the material in the fantasy comes from the unconscious. Thus the imaginal work enables us to contact material which has been unconscious and inaccessible. Not only can the new material transform us by producing more insight, it also causes bliss. The bliss is very important because it induces a non-dualistic state, devoid of a sense of time, of subject-object division, and of sensory functions.

Bliss states ocur all the time. They are not unusual or beyond our reach. However, they usually pass away, leaving us much as we were. What we learn through meditation is how to contact bliss and induce a state of timeless, non-dualistic unity. At first this is so pleasurable that it takes over the psyche as it has always done, but eventually we learn to maintain awareness of this as well and not be seduced into a trance-like state which leaves us with no recall. When we can retain awareness in the bliss state, we can utilize that bliss to activate the chakras.

BASIC SKILLS:
SPACIOUSNESS, CLARITY AND WARMTH

In imaginal work we seek meaning through symbolism. While symbolism is helpful, exclusive use of it can block access to deeper levels of meaning which are less symbolic and more experiential or feeling-toned. Spaciousness, clarity, and warmth can give us access to deeper meaning and more direct experience of the Inner Self. They are fundamental to all contemplative, meditative and imaginative activities.

Spaciousness

Spaciousness is the quality of openness and receptivity as well as attentiveness and mindfulness. When we employ spaciousness in our interactions with others, we are not just "open." When we are merely open, our minds may still be elsewhere. Even if we add attention, we still have mere attentiveness. With spaciousness, we are not only aware of all that is said, we also host a space which contains room for both parties to express their feelings without being locked into each other. When we become locked into a situation, for example when we are angry, we feel that the only remedy is to leave before the situation engulfs us. We have no choices. Spaciousness creates a space which is larger than the conscious interaction within which other possibilities and choices can manifest.

In Tibet, practitioners who were developing spaciousness traditionally went to the mountains. They would sit on a cliff which overlooked the sky, which, in Tibet, is often quite blue and clear. They would sit and watch its spaciousness. Usually we take the sky for granted, assuming it is limited and has boundaries like everything else. However, if we really look at the sky we will realize that it is expansive, infinite, of immeasurable depth. This realization produces a feeling of awesomeness which many describe as a numinous experience in itself. Thus, sitting and watching the sky, we experience its profundity. And we realize something else as well: the sky is really a mirror of our own psyche or mind.

Human consciousness is infinite, just like the sky. It contains all our thoughts, memories and perceptions. It is the greatest achievement of all creation. Thoughts appear in it like objects in the sky. When a bird flies through the sky it captures our attention. We forget the sky because we are preoccupied with the bird. It seems as if only the bird exists. The sky is non-existent because we are no longer aware of it. In the same way thoughts seize our attention constantly so that we are never aware of the mind in which they occur.

However, if we continue to watch the thought or the bird, we will see that eventually it disappears or sinks into the depths of the sky or mind, and what remains is the sky or the mind itself. Then the practitioner realizes that the mind is a huge expansive container, like the sky. Each thought, feeling and emotion arises in the mind, captures our attention for a moment, and, just like the bird, disappears or dissolves into the mind, leaving it as before.

Once the practitioner, watching the sky, sees how the bird mirrors his own psychic experiences, he experiences the contents of his psyche in a new way. For example, when he gets hungry he experiences the hunger, like an image of the bird, within the context of his psyche. If he maintains awareness of the spaciousness of his psyche, the hunger will often dissolve naturally into the spaciousness. Other thoughts and feelings will arise to replace it, but he has now realized that — just by staying with the hunger while maintaining awareness of the immense sky or psyche — the hunger will disappear on its own, just like the bird. The pattern of birds and clouds in the sky continues, just as thoughts and emotions do in the psyche, but they will disappear into the sky or mind without any effort.

When he can experience a thought and the expansiveness of the mind simultaneously, the practitioner realizes that he can accept things more easily if he does not project his own likes and dislikes onto the psychic content. Usually, our attention is determined by how much we like or dislike what occurs. If we don't like something, we avoid it. The unconscious consists of everything blocked by our avoidance. But if we like something, we try to hold onto it and extend its existence. That's how our psyche normally functions. However, once we learn to simply focus awareness on the emotion, thought or experience, our perception is no longer controlled by our dispositions, likes, dislikes and preconceptions. Normally, these factors determine our experience. When we can experience thought and emotion arising from the depths of the psyche, we can tolerate ugliness and cruelty because we know that they will disappear on their own.

But spaciousness is not simply important because it frees us from the tyranny of the likes and dislikes that determine our interaction with others and our day-to-day experience. The effort required to avoid what we dislike and pursue what we do like consumes most of our energy, so that we have no energy left to nurture our growth. Once we begin to live our

lives with spaciousness, our experiences are not so predeter-
mined by attraction and avoidance, and within the infinite
container of the psyche in which our thoughts and feelings
arise is spaciousness and the freedom to act as we choose.

Then, even when we do become angry, we no longer feel
like we are locked in a prison because now we can connect to
spaciousness. There we will find that there are many ways to
deal with anger besides lashing out. No matter how important
we feel our anger is, we know it is still just a part of the psyche.
This insight also enhances our imaginal work. If, when we
connect to a dream image and let it unfold, we lose awareness
of the spaciousness of the psyche, then the image may take
over our psyche and engulf us, involving us in the process of
projection. This limits the imaginal work and our ability to
benefit from it. Instead we need to just watch the image unfold,
like the practitioner watches the bird in the sky.

Clarity

The second skill is clarity. Clarity is experiencing what is
happening *as it is* rather than as it appears, without our projections. For example, if someone appears hostile, our tendency is to base our interaction on our perception of hostility;
thus we become defensive. If we develop clarity, we will be
able to see beyond the surface appearance of hostility to what
really *is*, and to base our interaction upon that. Because clarity
helps us tolerate someone's initial appearance, we say that it
pierces through everyday appearances to get at the truth like
a sword. Many mythic figures carry swords representing
discrimination or clarity, the ability to discriminate between
appearance and truth. We apply clarity in imaginal work by
looking beyond our initial perception of dream images to
discover the real image behind them.

Warmth

The third skill is warmth, a term which includes receptivity
and friendliness. When we interact with warmth, we are not
caught up in our intellect or fantasies. Instead we are warm,

open and engaged, so that we experience our own or the other person's every thought or feeling with receptivity and friendliness. When we apply this technique to ourselves, we will find that it is easier to own up to why we are experiencing particular thoughts and feelings if we approach them with warm receptivity.

When we have warmth, we can be warm towards someone even if we must say something that hurts him or her; we can also host unpleasant thoughts and feelings. When we have spaciousness and clarity we do not react automatically to a person or a thought. We can choose how we will respond.

Thus spaciousness, clarity, and warmth are the basic skills for transforming our relationships with other people and our own thoughts.

HOSTING THE PSYCHE

Before one attends to the contents and processes of the inner journey, the psyche needs to be hosted in a way that will allow one to carry on an intimate conversation with it. In order to engage in such a conversation, the psyche must be hosted in such a way as to facilitate the openness and authenticity that is crucial to the process of intimate conversation. One way to do this is to host the clinical encounter as a sacred space in which you can enter into an authentic mode of being. In fact, the clinic becomes a space wherein you may share your feelings, anxieties and hopes with an openness and wholeness hosted by the Inner Self. This is especially important for Westerners, for whom the greatest obstacle on the spiritual path is lack of familiarity with the psyche. Our knowledge of it is so poor that to us it is only a concept, an experience or feeling. Yet it is more than that. It is truly the greatest wonder in the world, because it contains all the information, experience, and feelings that exist or have ever existed. It is the creator of most of the world, including the technology that makes our lives so comfortable. It contains both our conscious and unconscious processes and hosts our many experiences over many lifetimes. So when we say that the psyche needs to be hosted, we mean that we need to acknowledge its sacredness. Because in the past we have failed to honor it as the source of all that we have and are, we have distanced ourselves from its reality as our spiritual essence, as the source of our spirituality which also contains our goal: the Inner Self. We need to honor and respect it because by it we are made or broken.

Here in the West we have no space in our houses for even a small representation of our most sacred inner selves. In fact, we have lost our connection to such an extent that we find it difficult even to understand how a statue or picture of a deity can represent the Inner Self. By way of contrast, even the poorest family in India or Tibet finds space in their shanty for an altar or shrine which symbolizes the psyche. There they honor it and create a connection to it.

To begin, we must make the gesture of honoring the Self by creating a space for it. This is how we announce to it and to ourselves that we have resolved to undertake the inner journey. Unless we create that sacred space, we cannot even begin.

Such a space may be created within the home, be it a whole room or just part of a room. This sacred space, which houses symbols of your Inner Self and objects of inspiration, becomes the place which you enter when you want to engage in intimate conversation with your psyche and its components. The place is sacred not because it is secret, something you hide from everyone else. It is sacred because it is a symbol of your own psyche that you can sense, feel, and experience and within which you can carry out a conversation without inhibition.

Since our shrine symbolizes our psyche — especially that part which speaks very deeply to us — we should place objects upon it which symbolize the Self. Traditionally that meant a statue of the Buddha, representing the body, though we should use something that represents our own bodies. Tibetans also place a Buddhist text on their shrine to represent speech, and a bell and scepter to represent the mind or psyche itself. We must select personal symbols to represent our minds, bodies and speech, the capacity and power they possess and which we want to tap. These will be different for each of us.

What is important is that they should be personally meaningful. It may take time to figure out what they are. That's okay. Our choices should be guided by how deeply they speak to us and also by how comfortable we feel with them because we will be conversing intimately with them.

These symbols create a temporary structure in which we can contact the Self. They help form a link between us and our true Self and also act as go-betweens. It is the act or ritual of setting up the shrine which informs the Self that we wish to contact it — unlike before, when we ignored it. We use this symbolic gesture to draw the Inner Self forth from the deep unconscious. Before the process is complete and the Self is completely drawn forth, we will work with many different symbols and experience their growth and transformation. In the end, when we finally do reach the Self, we will let go of all symbols.

As a part of hosting the psyche, the way we are present in the sacred space becomes a statement of our motivation and confidence in the process. Our physical posture and presence in the sacred space reflect our sincerity and authenticity in carrying out intimate conversation. An upright position in the room informs yourself and the world that you are encountering your psyche as honestly as you can.

If we have never honored or hosted the psyche, the source of spirituality, no temple or spiritual doctrine can fulfill us; these external symbols can only manifest what is within us. No church or temple can do what we can only do by ourselves: host the Inner Self. Once we have done so, then the church or spiritual doctrine can manifest it.

PRAYER: LISTENING TO THE DIVINE

For many of us, prayer is simply an act of supplicating the Divine for guidance. In spiritual work, however, we need to deepen our experience of prayer so that it can establish our connection or relationship with the Divine, which is itself a manifestation of the Inner Self. It is rarely addressed early in the spiritual path because so much of Western spiritual practice mimics a psychological, particularly Jungian, approach which focuses on hearing the Self alone. Consequently the Self becomes the focus of the spiritual process and little attention is paid to the notion of prayer, which develops out of a religious rather than a psychological context. By contrast, prayer attempts to contact a deity external to ourselves which is a projection of the Self. In the East, where spiritual development grew out of religious tradition, prayer is addressed more fully and used to deepen and enrich spiritual growth.

Effective use of prayer is important in any genuine spiritual practice because we must be able to hear the inner Self through the Divine. If we bypass it we will probably never hear the full potentials of the Self. So it is critical in the preliminary stages to establish a strong connection with the Self through the Divine. At the beginning we are like a newborn baby in relationship to the spiritual — totally helpless, unable to communicate or verbalize our needs. Thus we need to learn to invoke the spiritual and to build a sense of trust that it will respond to our needs. Prayer can establish this communication and bond us with the Divine.

Just as a baby is too unsophisticated to really express his needs and must trust the mother to understand and respond, so prayer is not primarily a *verbalization* of our personal needs. Instead, its essence is contained in four steps which will establish a connection with the Divine and the trust that our personal needs will be heard.

Evocation

The first step is evocation — evoking the Divine from our mind's spaciousness with clarity and warmth. Many of us only pray when we are in need; very few of us ever try to evoke. Instead we seek immediate connection with the Divine in the hope of receiving instant help. Evoking means to visualize an image of the Divinity in the spaciousness of our consciousness. There are many ways of doing this, whether in silence or by recitation of a prayer specifically designed to evoke the image.

Connecting to the Divine

After evocation, the next step is connecting to the Divine. Connection means feeling attuned with the Divine and acknowledging its presence once it is evoked. This kind of conscious acknowledgment of the relationship gives it credibility and substance, which not only strengthens the presence of the Divine, but increases the importance of our presence in the encounter.

Commitment

The third step is commitment, which, traditionally, is often presented as an offering, like the Buddhist mandala offering. Offering is a ritualized form of commitment. Commitment is important. Whenever we bring someone into our life, commitment solidifies the connection, giving it form and admitting responsibility by verbally acknowledging the relationship. The simplest form is saying "I love you," or perhaps giving or receiving a ring. Generally we commit to a relationship because we believe that it will foster our growth and well-being. The same dynamic needs to be enacted in our prayer.

Thanksgiving and Dedication

The last component of prayer is thanksgiving and dedication, which is how we acknowledge that the relationship with the Divine enriches our lives. We generate a sense of appreciation for the experience of connecting with the Divine as well as with others who reflect the Divine. It is also important in our relationships to develop the courage to acknowledge directly how they enrich us. Open acknowledgment of the value of a relationship permits it to grow by nurturing it at deep levels. It will make our prayer richer and deeper the next time. Offering thanksgiving for the relationship with Divinity makes it more likely that prayer will deepen into a naturally occuring process for us instead of something we do only in times of need.

Dedication means dedicating our experience to the welfare of people who are important to us, to all sentient beings, or to the planet. It establishes a connection between the very special, transcendent state that prayer has induced and our regular, mundane state of consciousness. Finding this connection is important for keeping the transcendent and the mundane from splitting off and becoming separate. If we can keep prayer from becoming merely a private experience which we do only at certain times and after which we move back into our daily routine, we can avoid experiencing our spirituality as something that only occurs in a certain frame of mind under certain circumstances at certain times, an experience which renders other events, times, or frames of mind mundane or ordinary rather than spiritual.

When we fail to connect our spirituality with the mundane world, we cannot spiritualize our relationships or the planet. One way of further nurturing the connection between the two is to constantly host even mundane experiences — like exchanges with other people and everyday emotions — with clarity, spaciousness and warmth, so that we cultivate them in everything we do or experience.

If we attempt to connect with the Divine simply by supplication or seeking guidance, we will fail to hear it because we are not open. Only when we can hear the Divine can it be hosted in our Inner Self, and only then can we hear what it really wants to say — rather than what we want it to say. Thus hosting the deity in silence, in the spirit of prayer, is one of the finest examples of prayer. To hear it is to form a connection with our own innner potentials or our Inner Self.

Prayer is also a process of asking. But the asking should be done by trusting the process of listening so that we don't have to verbalize the asking. We just trust the listening and the openness itself to contain the process of asking.

The actual form of our prayer may vary from a simple process of listening in silence to an elaborate ritual. Either type of prayer can be done as a preliminary to our main spiritual practice, meditation, contemplation, or any kind of self-actualizing practice — or it can be a complete spiritual practice in itself. When used in this latter form, prayer becomes the essence of all spiritual practice.

We are now ready to begin the actual process itself. Each step of the process is presented as a question which we must work through, not just intellectually but also emotionally and spiritually. Without all three kinds of insight we cannot advance on the spiritual path.

QUESTIONNAIRE: THE PATH TO DEPTH INNER WORK AND PERSONAL GROWTH

Preliminary Questions

1. What is it that makes me want to change and grow at this point in my life?

2. What capacity do I have to be with others in an authentic and loving way?

3. How far can I accept the realities and circumstances of life as an integral part of myself?

The Actual Path to Inner Work

1. When I am hurt, disappointed and lonely, what provides refuge from the hurt and loneliness?

2. How deeply am I committed to being with others, recognizing that my well-being is closely tied with their well-being?

3. What part of me needs to be initiated and empowered so that I can begin the ritual of growth and transformation?

4. What kind of mandala should I enter into which will provide the kind of environment that can facilitate an authentic way of being for growth to take place?

5. When do I know that I am getting fixated and stuck at a particular stage of growth, and how do I know that even as I journey into my inner world I am not fantasizing or letting my imagination disconnect from the reality of my being?

6. How do I host my imaginal work in an authentic way, and what do I need to do to enhance its ministrations, its voice and cooperative collaboration in my growth?

7. How will I know when the Inner Self is experienced and how can it be brought into the service of growth and development?

8. How do I actualize my imaginal work and the Inner Self in my daily living so that I can incorporate what they tell me into my experience?

9. How will the above processes and insights help me with my hurts and conflicts, as well as help me to mature and grow?

In working with these twelve stages, the following two questions should also be added to each of the above stages:

A: How will I and others close to me know that I have changed or am attempting to change at this point in my growth?

B: What am I likely to do that will frustrate the process of growth and development I am seeking?

These twelve steps are the basis of contemplative depth psychotherapy. Each step involves extensive insights and inner work processes. The inner journey is by no means a linear process, rather it is a spiraling or circular process in which each student must find his own bearings. Each student may begin at any one of the twelve stages, feeling free to stop and retrieve a thought or experience from the previous stage in order to move forward.

The purpose of the preliminary process is to assess the psyche's receptivity to the inner journey and determine our ability to perceive and intuit inner states, which is an essential skill. Through this process we will acquire a deeper understanding of ourselves.

RENUNCIATION

1. What is it that makes me want to change and grow at this point in my life?

In finding a centering point in the quest for inner experience, the first question which stages the backdrop for the unfoldment of your inner journey within your personal history of pain and joy, triumph and tribulation, is integral to honoring both your being as well as your aspirations to move forward. The question is:

What is happening in my life that makes me want to change?

This question corresponds to the traditional step called questioning and renunciation.

Since renunciation means different things to each of us, we need to determine its meaning for us personally. We also need to question our surface-level answers in order to evoke a deeper answer, which we do by exploring images and symbols which appeal to us. These will tell us more about our hidden, unconscious selves.

Basically, renunciation is a desire to change our way of being. Although traditionally it is viewed as a process of denial, it is really a process of letting go, of acknowledging old patterns and working with a process of wanting to change, even while knowing that we will not always be able to change fully or immediately. If we renounce only at the level of denial, simply by labeling our bad habits and pushing them away, we do not undergo authentic renunciation. Genuine renunciation involves exploring our dark, unconscious sides in order to discover what keeps us from changing. It begins with a simple willingness to hear this side of ourselves.

Initially, we are only willing to include light into our sacred space. However, we will gradually reach the point where we can renounce that which prevents us from hosting the dark. Without such authentic renunciation, unconscious figures cannot really be present. So renunciation involves learning new skills in order to learn more about who and what we are.

The first step is: we must learn more about what we want to renounce. We do not tire of the world and decide to begin the spiritual journey by chance. Something has occurred which has caused us to become dissatisfied with life. We need to identify that event in order to connect with our own myth.

For any breakthrough to take place in the inner journey, the event must have the capacity to move the soul in such a way that one is profoundly motivated towards inner work. Significant dreams, visions, spiritual experiences such as kundalini awakening, the loss of a loved one and so on are some of the events which people say make them want to explore personal growth and development. The questions, however, which need to be explored are: How deeply has the soul of the person really been moved by the event? and:

How does the individual experience and respond to the event?

If the event's significance manifests through symptoms of inflation, then clearly the soul is not moved in such a way that the client can effect a change at the level which inner work demands.

Inflation

Inflation makes one view his experience of a dream, kundalini awakening or whatever as a *total* experience in and of itself. Consequently, he or she projects interpretations upon it which far exceed reality. The experience of the event usurps the central position of the Inner Self and, due to its complete occupation of the psyche, makes it exceedingly difficult for the Inner Self to surface. Often it may lead to decisions that are abrupt and sudden, without taking into consideration the reality of the situation. This is a result of one's failure to host the significance *and* limitations of the experience. Any attempt to point out the person's projection will be met with resistance.

For the event to truly move an individual in a way that connects him to the inner journey, he must first fall from that state of inflation which exists in relationship to the event. Paradise must be given up so that he may leave the Garden of Eden and discover and reconcile himself with the true Self. The assumption that the event is a whole, the state of being at one with nature, the total identification with the event to the exclusion of reality, must be shattered in order to see through the mists of inflation. "In the state of alienation, the ego is not only disidentified from the Self, which is desirable, but is also disconnected from it, which is most undesirable."

Inflation culminates in alienation, which is a necessary prelude to awareness of the Inner Self. In fact, after an intense alienation experience which involves a complete absence of any sense of transpersonal support or foundation for one's existence to rest upon, a breakthrough usually occurs which leads the person to seek ways to fill the emptiness he feels. Edward Edinger says:

> "When inflation occurs the ego can be re-deemed only by restoring to the Self its lost honor. This, however, is not sufficient for full satisfaction. Grace derived from the Self's self-sacrifice must complete the payment. There is even the hint that the ego's inflation and subse-quent penalty are necessary to generate the flow of healing energy [grace]..."

The Example of the World's Great Teachers

All the myths of the world's great spiritual teachers record the event which provoked the awakening that caused the teacher to want to change. The event made the incipient world teacher realize that material life is a painful process which cannot answer all our questions. This questioning led these individuals to renounce the mundane world and its answers to life's problems.

Let us examine the story of the Buddha and see what made him want to change. He was born the son of a king, who of course wanted his son to succeed him. However, when an astrologer predicted that the prince would either be a great king or a spiritual teacher who would renounce the world, the king made every effort to shield the boy from pain and suffer-ing out of fear that he might be moved to give up his royalty and inheritance for the life of a renunciant. As fate would have it, one evening the young prince encountered a very sick, feeble man being helped along by his mother. The prince grew alarmed and asked his attendant what was wrong with the man. When his attendant told him, the prince asked if everyone, including himself, was subject to illness. And the attendant replied in the affirmative. In the next few days the young prince encountered an old man worn out by age, a procession carrying a dead body to the cremation grounds, and finally a monk who had renounced the world. For nights the prince struggled with these experiences and questioned himself. If the truth of life involved such experiences, how could one hide from them?

For the prince to individuate, he had to leave the state of inflation which palace life had nourished within him. The events, traumatic though they were, nevertheless created the opportunity for him to walk into the loneliness and the unknown with that courage which is necessary in order to sustain us through initial alienation and pain. Inner work demands that such an experience precede it because that is what life, with all its ups and downs, demands of us. And this is what we demand of our children and all those we love and care for.

The significance of an event that heralds the inner work is enhanced if it sparks a sense of connection to the collective nature of such an experience. In some ways we, in experiencing the need to change, host the sensations that allow us to savor what the great spiritual teachers also experienced. In this potential we are presented with a sense of bonding, and thus a kind of lineage is created. It is this collective experience of the event that allows us to move forward towards the individuation process.

Self-Knowledge and Emptiness

And yet the desire for freedom is not, in and of itself, enough. To progress on the path to freedom we must also understand ourselves and our motivations more deeply. We begin by evoking a deeper resonance within us to the event which made us dissatisfied with the world and its answers.

So when the world and its answers no longer satisfy us and we decide to seek out different ones, we must assess our capacity to seek out new answers. This is the second part of the first step. None of us are foolish enough to begin a physical journey without carefully packing our bags and checking to make sure we have everything we need. We need to do the same before beginning our spiritual journey.

In exploring our own motivations for renunciation we mimic the patterns of the great teachers and generate confidence in ourselves. Confidence becomes important when we begin to use imaginative fantasy, emotions and feelings in our spiritual practice. Confidence helps us trust the process. If we do not have it, the life experiences which evoke emotions of failure, suffering and fear will bring our journey to a halt because we will give up.

So it is not enough to have had a traumatic event or spiritual experience or to have become fed up with the material world or curious about spiritual experience, or even to search for the meaning of life. All these reasons come from places of need. Renunciation is more than a desire to escape suffering or boredom or to deepen our devotion. Many of us do start on the spiritual path for these reasons; however, in order to continue we must explore beneath the surface level and infuse our stance with greater depth and feeling.

What we bring to the path is the totality of our life experience, all our sadness, joys, trials, triumphs and tragedies. Deep renunciation requires more than rational, analytical expression about an emotional crisis which causes us to want change. This only involves psychic content, not the psyche itself — which, after all, is the part of ourselves which has actually had the experience. For true renunciation to occur, the psyche itself must change or shift.

To evoke such a shift, connect with the story of a great teacher whose tale of renunciation has moved you deeply. It doesn't matter what religion the teacher represents. What we are seeking is *resonance*. If the story deeply arouses our emotions, it will evoke images and fantasies. We should explore and play with these images. It is a mistake to leave the story at a cognitive level. We must let it vibrate or strike a chord in our hearts.

What does striking a chord mean? It doesn't mean that we have a big emotional experience. It means that movement occurs, as when the resonance of a single note produces a chord. In its moving it generates images, memories, fantasies, and produces bliss. We should go with these experiences because, no matter how childish or irrelevant they may seem to be, they are enormously significant because they arise from the unconscious. Thus we have connected with and evoked the unconscious, the great unknown.

If what is evoked for us is emotion, we don't let it overwhelm us so that we release it, for this dissipates the energy. Instead of dissipating the feeling, we contain and experience it so that it produces more images and more psychic energy. The generation of psychic energy is really the key to the Tantric process. If we practice this technique whenever we have a spiritual experience, the images will produce new psychic energy. Then we can use the energy to produce more experience. If we do not evoke more feeling by following the images, we remain on the cognitive level, new energy doesn't arise, the energy dissipates, the feeling goes, and we have gotten nowhere.

Besides teaching us how to do Tantric imaginal work, this exercise deepens our renunciation by revealing to us some unconscious aspects of it. We get to know ourselves better. As we deepen our experience of ourselves, we discover new parts, like our intuition, our spirituality, our mythic selves. These in turn help us communicate with even more mystical internal experience. However, it is important to understand that it is not just the content of experience that measures or determines our spiritual process, but rather the psychic state. The ability to connect with deeper levels is what differentiates working with material on a spiritual level as opposed to the psychological or religious. We need to learn to shift into different states of consciousness so that we can experience material in a variety of ways, not just through a devotional, analytical awestruck or emotive perspective.

The ability to trust the image or symbol sufficiently to allow it to shift into deeper states is pliancy of mind. As we said before, it is a fundamental skill to use in combating fixed ways of intepreting spiritual experience and minimizing attachment to new experience. It takes on deeper meaning because we use the entire multifaceted psyche to contain experience and to view it from different perspectives.

As we examine our spiritual experience and assess our abilities, we must determine how much of the range of human experience we appreciate. In other words, we must get a sense of how much of ourselves we are conscious of. Do we see ourselves as biological, cognitive, thinking persons functioning on cognitive, goal-oriented or structure-defined levels? Do we validate our feelings and our intuitive experiences as well? How do we handle events that are not rationally explainable, such as synchronistic events? Are we comfortable with the images that may arise in us when we meet a person?

If we only feel comfortable in a cognitively defined universe, we are locking out large portions of ourselves which we cannot authenticate or of which we cannot possibly even admit the existence. However, to be well prepared for our journey we must acknowledge the existence of deep states beyond even feelings and intuitions and feel ourselves to be participants in a larger process of human experience. We need to be open to these parts of ourselves because, on the journey, it is through these faculties that we will progress.

To explore these, we must renounce old behavior patterns, thinking processes, and emotions which block our growth. Some of us must do psychological work to overcome childhood issues or problems with aggression or fear.

How do we handle synchronistic, illogical, out-of-context, contradictory events? Frequently we have little tolerance for such things and dismiss them as irrational and irrelevant. Or we trivialize them by explaining them away, or refuse to admit they even exist. However, acknowledgment of and tolerance for the irrational is required, because the psyche contains everything. Since the purpose of inner growth is to consciously integrate all of its sides into a multi-dimensional form, we must deepen our sense of wholeness, of totality.

Also, we need tolerance for transitoriness or emptiness. Most of us fear emptiness; we call it "existential anguish". To avoid the terror of death or emptiness, we refuse to confront it, a tactic which produces self-involved, self-generating, self-perpetuating narcissism. In our total involvement with avoiding the terror of death and emptiness, we function entirely from an "I need" place. We are so deeply involved in this that it sounds perfectly normal! However, to begin the spiritual journey we must be willing to confront our fear of emptiness, death and change, and this means that we must be willing to let go of needs-based psychology. Otherwise we will never reach our goal or even begin our journey.

This is so important that Buddhists train to learn to tolerate emptiness. Eventually we must not only tolerate it but learn to create images in the emptiness. They differ from the images that normally appear to us because they are consciously produced rather than created unconsciously from fears and projections.

Finally the spiritual practice involves not only deepening our capacity for internal experience, but actualizing our inner growth in our interactions with others. This is the greatest spiritual practitioner: the one who returns to the world and measures the worth of his internal spiritual experience by his capacity to reflect it in his interaction with others.

BEING WITH OTHERS COMPASSIONATELY

2. What capacity do I have to be with others in an authentic and loving way?

The second question of the preliminary process is: what capacity do we have to be with others authentically? Many people do not expect to do this when doing inner spiritual work. In many spiritual traditions it is enough to go off to a mountain top and have spiritual experiences. Even some types of Buddhism have as their goal the attainment of purely individual liberation. However, the Mahayana tradition believes that a capacity to be with others is a fundamental requirement in the spiritual process, without which we cannot embark on the path.

Frequently, the event that has caused us to want to change has also made us feel alienated and distant, misunderstood and lonely. It may have isolated us because we could not share it with others. As a result, we may feel lost in darkness. This feeling may bring us to a standstill at the very start. To move beyond this standstill we must be able to access our inner strength or find strength in others. This is so important that our capacity to do so determines our capacity for spiritual growth, because throughout our journey we will constantly encounter loneliness and pain. We need to be able to access inner reserves of strength in order to continue. So we need to explore our capacity to be with others — not just out of love for others, but out of love for ourselves as well, for the quality of our being with others is a test of our inner selves.

At this point what we need to do is assess our current capacities for sharing our inner experience with others and for allowing others to nourish us.

Let us look at how we bring spirituality into our interaction with others. Our culture says that a statement like the following one is healthy: "I am very angry with you for not closing the door." It says that this is healthy because we are expressing our emotion toward the other person. However, if we examine our body language and the content of our words, we will realize that they have a demanding, critical quality, particularly if these are supported by our tone of voice.

What is criticism? It has four components: an emotion, an external event, a judgment, and a demand. The emotion, of course, is anger. The event, in this case, is not closing the door, which causes the anger. The judgment is: "You are a bad person for doing that." The implied demand is: "Don't do it next time."

Though most of us have been taught that this is an acceptable way to relate to others, we can relate more empathetically if we are willing to look beyond the superficiality of this kind of statement. If we can hear the demand and the judgment, we can see that the person making this statement is only in touch with his or her masculine, shadow side. Even the light side of the masculine is not present — only the demanding, angry side of the dark side of the masculine. It is certainly not in touch with the feminine.

In this five-second encounter in which the person manifests himself, we can judge him as he does us: "This person is a very bad person. He's inconsiderate and he's angry at me." It is hard to resist the impulse to react by feeling mistreated, abused, and threatened, and wanting to respond from our own dark masculine side. But a more spiritual way to react is to recognize that the other person is coming from *his* dark masculine side, and so react more empathetically and with less judgment. We can do this only if we develop awareness.

When we have awareness, we have choice. So we may choose in this case to experience anger or whatever reaction we feel, but not release it. If we have a sense of spaciousness, then we can deal with the person more empathetically. Though we feel angry, we do not let that anger engulf us and so cause us to release it unempathetically by saying: "I am very angry with you. You said this and I feel very angry." Spaciousness and clarity help us sense, beyond the offensive words, the innate good feeling which the other person contains as well.

So speaking our needs and expressing our feelings may restrict us to a superficial level of response, because underneath the surface emotion are several deeper levels of feelings. If we can become conscious of these, we can begin to resonate at deeper levels in our relationships. Then, when someone forgets our birthday, we will sense that beneath our anger we feel unloved and uncared for. Underneath these feelings are other feelings of unimportance and unworthiness. We need to work towards sharing the deeper feelings, not just the surfaces.

Meditation is a good way to train ourselves in skills with which to enhance relationships; however, unless we practice with people, our meditative skills will reach a point after which they will not grow. If we integrate them into real life, then the meditative practices will evolve to a much finer level.

In working with others, we are frequently taught that unconditional love is the greatest love we can offer another. However, authentic empathy goes a step further because it not only wishes the other person well but actively wishes that he or she shall not suffer. We also need discrimination to really help others. To love wisely, we must use wisdom as the basis of unconditional love. Frequently, we think love has no limits; however, its expression is limited or conditioned by our ability to use it wisely. For example, when someone is hurting us it is not the time to practice unconditional love! Actually, it is conditioned because, since we have left the meditative state and returned to the relative world, we too are conditioned by events. The final test of our love is to be in the state of bliss and, though we want to share it, to be sensitive to the other person and willing to operate on his or her level. Thus we do not impose our unconditional love on others.

If someone is bullying us, we can nevertheless generate unconditonal love towards him while tempering its expression with discrimination. If we do not, we may express love in an unskillful manner so that we are unfairly treated. So we might use assertive behavior to contain the bully and prevent more destructive beahvior.

Using these five guidelines, we can manifest unconditional love. Without them, we cannot share our experience of unconditonal love and we will experience the outer world as frustrating. For example, if we lack discrimination in our practice of unconditional love we will be taken advantage of, or if we do not take the right action to contain violence either we ourselves or the other person may be harmed. This touches on an important difference between the Buddhist practice of unconditional love and that which is characteristic of other groups. We maintain that if our motivation is concern for the other person, then even if, in aggressive or assertive situations, we must resort to strong language or behavior that is unpleasant and is experienced as such by the other person, we are still acting from love.

In addition, unfocused unconditional love which lacks the meditative skills of concentration and attention is draining. Without focus, our unconditional love remains an unfocused, panoramic experience, enjoyable to ourselves but hardly practical or of use in the real world.

UNDERSTANDING THINGS AS THEY ARE IN-STEAD OF AS WE WISH THEM TO BE

3. How far can I accept the realities and circumstances of life as an integral part of myself?

The third and last step of the preliminaries asks us to determine whether or not we are able to accept the realities and circumstances of life as an integral part of living.

In this step we continue to work to integrate our spiritual lives with our humanity and to live our lives as part of a spiritual process. It involves giving up many of our notions about the world and accepting it as it really is. It completes the preliminary process because, having hosted the Inner Self, reached a point where we want to change, and having evaluated our capacity to be with others, we now explore how to accomplish these goals, based on reality. To live in a real way means to accept the world's reality.

But first we must define wisdom and living wisely. Buddhists define wisdom in terms of the principle of truth, maintaining that in the end it is truth that sets us free. Truth demands that we be true to whatever space we are in. This means that if we are hurt or in pain or grief, we must acknowledge that. Only then are we able to determine how to be wisely compassionate in situations in which we would otherwise go astray and be engulfed, or fail to be truly compassionate. Also, truth is not based solely on our own needs. We must also incorporate the collective truth or law of the cosmos and the soil.

One of these is the cosmic law of interdependence, which governs our lives. Due to it, we cannot merely express unconditional love because, due to our interdependence, we must respect others' boundaries. To flow with interconnectedness, we need truth or wisdom so that we can determine the most appropriate way to manifest our love. And since each of us is unique, we have to find our own way of being in the world, based on what is true for us at this time.

When we have answered the second question, there is a hint that the moment of truth has come. Now we must bring it into our consciousness and awareness. If we fail now to evaluate and make sense of our lives, we will have moments of inner insight, but always fall back into the old patterns. This will dishearten us and destroy our enthusiasm. We will suffer the pain of learning that, because we have not been truthful, the spiritual journey will have its ups and downs.

Among the monks whom the Buddha accepted as one of his followers was a very old monk with a very low I.Q. He was so stupid that he couldn't even learn the basic teachings; his memory was very poor and he couldn't remember anything. Because of this, the other monks rejected him. When the Buddha heard about this, he himself accepted the monk and taught him two simple phrases. Then he explained: "It is true that you are not in a position to benefit from the classes we run on spiritual work, so what I suggest is that you stay out. When the monks go in, they leave their shoes outside. Take a duster and clean their shoes and say your lines." The monk did this and was content. After several years, he discovered the meaning behind the simple practice, and, connecting to the truth, he attained inner realization. Then some nuns requested a teacher, and Buddha appointed this monk. The nuns were quite insulted, but since they could not reject him outright, they made a high platform for him to sit on, but one without stairs. This was in order to expose and ridicule him. However, when he came, the monk levitated up to the seat and gave various teachings. As he did so, the Buddha and his group passed by; satisfied, he moved on to the next village.

Here we see that the moment of truth had come for the monk and the nuns, as well as for the Buddha. The monk's moment of truth was declaring his realization. That of the nuns was transcending their superficial, collective concept of the monk. And the Buddha's was in realizing that these moments had come and that it was time for him to leave the monk to honor his own truth. Also, this story shows that we can reach the numinous without going through the intellectual. Similarly, we all have to discover the moments in our lives when the truth as a revealing source will set us free. We may feel that truth comes in meditation, though in fact the spiritual experience alone is not sufficient for us to honor ourselves. Our potential is even greater. And we must be able to hear that moment of truth.

If we confine our spiritual practice to a wise, safe, cognitive, analytical, intellectual level, we may miss the moment of truth that comes to hint that our potential is much greater.

That which sets us free is something we must find for ourselves. There is no collective truth which will tell us what that is. We must each find it for ourselves. We must begin to listen for it constantly, because spiritual work is not just about meditating or cultivating love or being calm and tranquil. The truth of the universe, of the soil which feeds us, of the cosmic laws which govern nature, are the truths which we must hear resonating in our spirituality. Insofar as we do so, the spark of freedom will appear, and our numinous experiences will take on a greater inner worth. We need to make truth the guiding light in all our experiences, including our emotions and relationships. If we practice in this way, then wisdom will come because it always comes when truth is the basis.

The Tibetan tradition identifies three types of wisdom or truth which we must embody: personal truth, collective truth, and universal truth.

The wisdom of personal truth is wisdom of who we are. As we have seen, the initial work of this process lies in cultivating wisdom and determining who and where we are right now. This determines how we can use truth to set ourselves free and what the moment of truth means for us. It involves acquiring a sense of the self, a term which includes the ego, the self and the inner Self. The small self is the totality of all that we, as individuals, are composed of: our bodies, sensory experiences, emotions, cognitions. The ego is what helps the self interact with the environment. The Inner Self lies deep in our psyches and is usually unavailable to us. Generally, we are too caught up in the environment and in our struggle to maintain balance and sanity between the environment and ourselves. So the Inner Self regresses or is hidden.

We need to get a sense of each level of the self. One way to sense the ego is to recollect an extremely intense emotional experience, like intense anger, and become aware of how we experience ourselves. After meditating for a while, we will see that the ego is grasping.

The self is a collection of parts that make up a whole, and so it cannot be identified as this or that — unlike the more concrete ego. It never tends to be experienced except as a philosophical or religious concept. However, we need to get a sense of the difference between acting from our egos and from the self, because we instinctively tend to believe that the self and the ego are the same, although this is a denial of the truth. In fact, this is the primordial cause of denial, repudiating truth at a very primol level.

It is important to acquire a sense of the ego as opposed to the self, a person who is a foundation for hosting the truth — for unless we know what is true, how can truth set us free? We must know the difference between our self as a person, and our self which interacts with others, i.e. the persona. Who we are as a person is determined by collective cosmic law, but how we interact with others is determined by the ego. The self connects us to other people, other selves in this universe, and to the ability to experience them not just as angry or bad people but as individuals composed of many units: body, mind, emotions, thoughts and fears. When we relate to someone through the self we relate to a complex being. At the ego level our actions, feelings and interactions with others are determined by our fears, jealousies, injuries, psycho-sexual or aggressive drives, by our own needs — so that any connection with the *other* is severed. When we relate to others through the self we can form connections between our different parts.

The third wisdom is most important. It is an inner wisdom which lives in a very wise part of us. In the East we have the myth of the spiritual warrior who lives in the spiritual, who is bound by truth. He does not kill his enemy deceptively. He has the courage to leave what is impossible to obtain, and to return when he is ready. We need this quality in our spiritual work today.

It is important to hear both the collective and the individual wisdom. Within us are many collective possessions — love, compassion, hatred, anger. These experiences are the same for all of us. Only the events that evoke them and the way we react to them are different. It is so with wisdom, in that it has a part which is collective and that all humanity shares, and an individual part. We need to find the collective treasure house of wisdom which includes the wisdom of both East and West, to connect to it so that it can serve as our guide, and then to share it with others.

10
REJUVENATION
THERAPY

INTRODUCTION

For centuries, people all over the world have been fascinated by the possibility of attaining youth and delaying the aging process. Everything from ancient rites and rituals to herbal treatments, modern cosmetics and surgery continue to be used by large numbers of people. The amount of money that is spent in the United States alone on youth and beauty products is astronomical, and although most of them are not scientifically proven they are in increasingly high demand. Is it possible to remain young by delaying the aging process? According to Tibetan medical literature, the answer is: Yes it is, but not by simply applying cosmetics or engaging in a sophisticated herbal treatment.

Rejuvenation, according to Tibetan medicine, means to rejuvenate one's mind, body and spirit. To do this, one has to work on all three of these levels, using appropriate techniques. For rejuvenation of the body, special herbal massage, herbal hydrotherapy, and herbal detoxification treatments are used. For revitalizing and developing the psycho-spiritual needs of the person, meditation, Yantra Yoga, and Buddhist growth and developmental techniques are recommended. When done under controlled conditions for the specified period of time, these programs produce positive results.

For centuries, Tibetan yogis and practitioners have been using the program as a part of their spiritual growth and development. They realized that in order to practice visualization and energy transformation processes, their minds and bodies had to be in peak performance states. Even in contemporary times, leading Tibetan teachers engage in this program, and there are accounts of lamas who were eighty years old or more and who looked extremely healthy and youthful — a rare occurrence in Tibet, where the average life span is forty-five years.

The rejuvenation program can be designed for different time periods depending on the person and what he wants to achieve. For instance, there can be a three-month or a one-year program. In the West, it is exceedingly difficult to do the full program according to the requirements set forth in the medical rejuvenation literature. This is because one is required to be away from daily stress and strain for the entire period of the program in an idyllic health resort far away from the city. To introduce the program to the West, a modified version will be described here. This program was first tried out in the summer of 1987 in Tuscany, Italy, by thirty Italian and Swiss partici-pants, and was extremely successful. The best part of the health resort was the cooperation of the managers, who appre-ciated and fully understood the need for quiet and contempla-tion during the entire period. Not only was the environment right, the spirit and energy at the center was healing and supportive.

REJUVENATION THERAPY

The program consists of two stages, a purification period that involves cleansing and detoxification, followed by reju-venation therapy which relies largely upon herbal prepara-tions.

The purification period is conducted for eight days in an idyllic, scenic and pleasant health resort, away from the noise and stress of the city. It is mandatory for all participants to complete this stage in order to cleanse, detoxify, organize an appropriate health plan in terms of nutrition, behavior, exer-cise, meditation and spiritual growth, as well as to learn how to conduct the rejuvenation therapy stage properly. The sec-ond stage is done during one's normal life and work and involves the regular use of an herbal rejuvenation pill for a period of three months.

What is the aim of this condensed rejuvenation program? No claim is being made that miraculous results will be obtained, since this is a modified and shortened program. However, it is designed to suit the time commitments of participants in the West and at the same time provide maximum benefits. During the 98 days, the program will infuse the individual with a sense of renewed energy and power, revitalize his skin and muscles, and improve his complexion and vital body functions such as digestion, blood flow, and nervous system activity. In short, this program is a physical and health promotion effort through treatment, education, and spiritual practice.

The Eight-Day Purification Period

The following daily routine must be followed by all participants for the first eight days of the program. This is a mandatory part of the rejuvenation program as it is essential to the effectiveness of the rejuvenation therapy. The details of the routine will be explained later.

7:00 A.M.   Wake up and bathe, rinsing your eyes with cold water and cleaning and massaging your tongue and gums. Evacuate bowels and bladder. In case of difficulty, take three glasses of cold water immediately after waking each morning until your bowel movements have been regulated.

7:30 A.M.   Drink a cup of nettle tea and then do meditation and Yantra Yoga.

8:15 A.M.   Have a breakfast of whole foods such as cereals, breads, fruits and herbal teas. Eat no meat or eggs.

9:00 A.M.   Hydrotherapy.

10:00 A.M.   Massage.

12:30 P.M.   Eat a vegetarian lunch.

2:30 P.M.	Medical examination, personality evaluation, and education.
4:30 P.M.	Yantra Yoga.
7:00 P.M.	Vegetarian dinner, with chicken and fish also available.
8:45 P.M.	Meditation.
10:30 P.M.	Sleep.

Cleansing the Body

One of the main features of holistic medicine, and one which is especially emphasized in the Tibetan tradition, is the need to detoxify the body before any major herbal or other form of treatment is prescribed. If toxins in the body are not removed, the treatment, no matter how effective, is severely limited, since the toxins prevent the herbs from working on the body. The first thing, therefore, is to cleanse the body. This can be done at various levels. During the first three days, regular hydrotherapy sessions are recommended, primarily to cleanse the skin, help the blood to flow more efficiently, and improve endocrine and secretory activity.

The bath therapy is especially effective with the use of the five nectar herbal formulae. These five herbal combinations work very effectively and may be used in liquid, crude or in pack form during the bath. In order to stimulate the healing powers of the herbs, light massage is recommended. The duration of the baths should be fifteen to twenty minutes for the first day, increasing gradually to 30 or 45 minutes during the next days. It is equally important to ensure that the water temperature is maintained, and if the water begins to cool the bath should be terminated.

If an individual has specific complaints such as joint pains or skin problems or would like to improve his or her skin complexion, special herbs are added to the five nectars. For instance, in order to improve the complexion, a variety of dried non-toxic flowers such as rose, jasmine and so forth are added to the base preparation. The baths in such cases are not only cleansing, they are therapeutic and can help to relieve symptoms such as chronic joint pains, skin conditions, etc.

In Tuscany, Italy, where the first program was held, there are several excellent natural hot springs which were ideal for the hydrotherapy sessions. Since such spots are public facilities, plastic and rubber bath tubes were used to collect the spring water for herbal baths. In Tuscany we also arranged sweat lodges in which small numbers of people participated, using herbal steaming as an alternative to herbal baths.

After the bath, 30 to 45 minutes of full body oil massage is recommended in order to clean toxins from the lymph nodes and stimulate blood circulation and other vital body functions. Oils and special herbal lotions help to improve skin complexion as well as muscle tone and activity. After the massage, acupressure is recommended in order to stimulate the flow of chi or energy in the body as well as help with specific complaints the participant may have. For instance, if the participant suffers from chronic low back pain, a special herbal medicated oil is applied both on the area of pain and discomfort and on the acupressure points. Then massage and acupressure are applied in order to help with the client's complaint so that he or she can carry out the rest of the program more efficiently.

The technique of full body oil massage comes from India and consists primarily of kneading, rubbing and stroking, or the application of an oil or lotion on the body. Muscular and fleshy parts of the body are kneaded while the rest of the body is rubbed vigorously, working towards the heart. The head and the abdomen are the two most important parts of the body which need to be worked on thoroughly — the head because it contains important acupressure points related to the chakras, and the abdomen because the metabolic or energy center is located here and the agni or digestive fire needs to be stimulated in order to keep the body healthy and active. Every session of massage requires careful work on these two areas.

After the massage, the participant is required to keep warm and, after 15 minutes, chickpea flour is applied to wipe away the oil or lotion. The purpose of this procedure is to fight the excess release of toxins into the blood stream which makes the client dull as a result of excess phlegm (Bagan) in the body. The chickpea flour dries away excess fluids and makes the blood flow to the skin as well as working to improve skin complexion and elasticity. After half an hour, the participant may wash off the chickpea powder.

In the early afternoons of the first three days, the participants will each be medically examined and take part in a personality and health test. However, before the personality test is carried out, each client is medically examined for any health complaints. If there are any imbalances, the participant is required to take herbal treatment for the next two days while continuing to take part in the eight-day program. It is crucial that the client should be in an optimal state of health during the eight days, and it is the physician's job to ensure that this is the case.

Internal Cleansing and Detoxification

Internal cleansing is absolutely essential in order for the body to be able to absorb the rejuvenating herbal preparations effectively. Before an internal cleansing is done, however, the participant is required to take a teaspoon of melted clarified butter before breakfast for three days, starting on the fourth day of the program. The purpose of taking the clarified butter is twofold: first, to activate toxins in the secretory and endocrine systems and localize them in the gastro-intestinal region for easy elimination via the rectum; and second, to lubricate the gastro-intestinal region in order to prevent the purgatives from irritating the linings of that area.

On the seventh day of the program, the participants are required to take a mild purgative first, and then later in the afternoon a stronger one in order to cleanse the gastro-intestinal region of all accumulated toxins. During the day, most of the routine program is curtailed in order to carry out the cleansing properly and efficiently. For certain participants, stronger purges may be necessary before they are cleansed. For others, a mild purge may do the job.

The eighth day is primarily spent in teaching the group about how to conduct the ninety days of rejuvenation therapy when they get back home. Classes in meditation and visualization of the Medicine Buddha are taught in detail. Following this, the ninety days supply of rejuvenation pills are distributed with instructions on how to take them.

Nutrition and Behavior

Nutrition during the eight-day program consists primarily of a vegetarian diet, with poultry and fish available for those who require animal protein. Participants are free to include any other food items they require. However, the following types of food are generally discouraged:

- white rice and white bread
- excess salads and raw vegetables belonging to the nightshade family, such as tomatoes, potatoes, eggplant, cabbage, etc.
- acidic, sour and fermented food items such as blue cheese, strong concentrated vinegar, miso, high acid producing food, spicy and greasy foods
- fatty foods such as mutton, beef and pork
- white refined sugar (fresh honey is permitted)
- ice cream, chocolate
- fresh, ripe fruits
- strong black tea or coffee
- carbonated drinks and alcohol

Breakfast is one of the most important meals and should consist of fruits, cereals, milk and brown bread. These should be heated if possible, since cold food is extremely hard on the body. If cheese is used, it is better to heat it and then apply it to bread or other food items. Lunch should include green vegetables, either in the form of stew or simply steamed with digestives such as ginger, cardamom or coriander. Brown rice should be well cooked but should not be washed too often. As brown rice is heavier than white, it is recommended that turmeric or garlic be mixed with it in order to help with digestion. Bread should be well baked and fresh. Heavy food and dairy such as cheese or butter should be taken heated, either with rice or bread. No high-sugar content food such as ice cream or chocolate is permitted. To get the sugar you need, fruits or recommended with honey or brown sugar. For dinner, a vegetarian meal with spinach or broccoli soup is recommended. For those who wish to take poultry or fish, the important thing is to prepare the dish in the proper way. Prepare these products in unsaturated fat and add condiments such as cumin, ginger, garlic and so forth. Fats should be removed from the chicken.

Any form of alcohol is prohibited, though medicinal wine may be permitted and even recommended for certain participants. Caffeinated beverages are not recommended, though decaffeinated tea or coffee may be taken with milk. During the day, nettle tea is recommended as an excellent cleanser and diuretic. Milarepa, the famous saint of Tibet, chose nettles as his main nutrition when he went into seclusion.

Equally important is the way you prepare your meals. For instance, there is no restriction if you cook the members of the nightshade family and mix them with protein items and add condiments. Similarly, gas and phlegm producing items like peas and beans lose these properties if they are well cooked and digestive aids added. In fact, when you have a heavy meal it is normally recommended that you drink a glass of hot ginger tea with honey immediately afterwards.

The time at which you eat your meals plays an important role. For instance, skipping breakfast or eating only a light breakfast is unhealthy for a Air (Lung) type, while for a Water (Bagan) type it is necessary to eat only a light breakfast. This is because Water is constitutionally most active during the morning, and eating a heavy meal will induce lethargy and dullness in a Water type. Similarly, if a Fire (Tripa) type eats a heavy protein lunch after 12:00 noon, he may experience nausea, headaches and fatigue as a result, because Fire is most active in the afternoon.

In general, any activity which induces stress, emotional distress and trauma is not recommended. Sex should be avoided during this period, as should any recall of painful memories. In short, the participant should do everything possible to fully enjoy the spirit and benefits of the eight-day program.

YANTRA YOGA

Yantra Yoga is an ancient Buddhist form of exercise that involves breathing, movement and concentration simultaneously. There are about seventy-five Yantra Yoga exercises, and during the program only the initial preparatory exercises are practiced. These include self-massage techniques using the fists and soles of the feet to apply sesame oil and massage oneself. After this, three different groups of preparatory exercises are taught and practiced regularly to coordinate breathing, movement and concentration. The whole purpose of Yantra Yoga is to help a person expend as little of his energy as possible in order to carry out a specific mental and physical activity. The core aim of a healthy practitioner is to be able to conserve as much energy as possible in the form of bodily heat, breath, and muscle use. By conserving these sources of energy, one's life span is increased as well as channeled towards higher purposes such as spiritual practice.

Yantra Yoga originated in the Indian system of Hatha Yoga and Tibetan yogis have used these exercises for centuries in order to keep themselves in peak physical and psychological condition. Having severed almost all contact with society, a yogi had to know how to take care of himself. To do so meant not only knowing about illnesses, their causes and treatments, but about the body in general, how it functions and how to keep it in good shape. Yantra Yoga, apart from its actual form (which involves spiritual practice), is designed to meet health needs and to assist the yogi in staying centered and grounded. What is clearly lacking among many practitioners of spirituality and meditation, especially in the West, is the concern and care that is needed for physical health and the sound perceptive and emotional organization which are important features in all spiritual practice.

During the program, it is mandatory for all participants to do an hour of Yantra Yoga every day. In cases of individual difficulties, the exercises can be modified to suit the individual. Yantra Yoga is indeed an important part of the program, as it gives the participant an holistic overview of himself and assists him in relating himself more efficiently to his internal and external experiences.

The meditational practices require faith, commitment, and regularity, as well as initiation. Since the entire practice cannot be described to those who have not undergone the initiation, an outline follows, using the Rejuvenation Meditation Thanka to help illustrate the process (see Illustration). Thanka is a Tibetan scroll painting.

THE THANKA DEPICTS FOUR MAJOR COMPONENTS OF THE PRACTICE:

1. Advantages in engaging in the practice
2. The site wherein practice takes place; the nature and quality of the environment; the behavioral compliances to observe
3. Actualizing the Rejuvenating and Healing Medicine Buddha in the form of the Five Dhyani Buddhas
4. The actual visualization and meditational practice

Advantages of Engaging in the Practice

- helps to increase one's life span by rejuvenating the mind and body
- prevents illness and mental negativity
- improves skin complexion, body energy and muscle tone
- improves sensory functions, memory and voice tone

Site, Environment and Behavior

- Observe the upper left hand portion of the Tanka, which depicts the following:
- the site where one practices should be clean, pollution free and isolated, but safe

- the environment should be scenic and natural, with abundant plants, herbs and water (see section 1)
- behavioral compliances involve the following:
- avoidance of extreme exposure to heat such as direct sunlight or fire (sections 2 and 3)
- avoid sex (section 4)
- avoid strenuous physical activities (section 5)
- the sensory and mental functions of the individual should be healthy (section 6)
- the individual should not be seriously ill or weak (section 7)
- the individual should not be suffering from severe mental ill health (section 8)
- the individual should not be over seventy years old (section 9)
- fermented, sour, acidic, heavy, raw food, or excessive intake of light green vegetables and salty food should be avoided (sections 10 through 14)
- an herbal bath should be taken before engaging in the meditational practice (sections 15 and 16)
- the herbal bath should be followed by an oleation and massage treatment, followed by an internal cleansing with purgatives (section 17)
- after the treatment, the individual becomes as strong, healthy and young as the animals depicted in the illustrations (sections 18 and 19)

Actualizing the Rejuvenating and Healing Medicine Buddha

After making sure that the herbs to be taken are placed in a clean container on a table in front of you, begin the practice of actualizing the Healing Buddhas as follows:

- Take refuge in the Guru, Buddha, Dharma and Sangha.
- Take the Bodhisattva Vow of altruism.
- Create the appearance of the Medicine Buddha in the space in front of you.

- Dissolve your ordinary self into emptiness from which you appear as a healing deity such as Vajrapani.
- Visualize in front of you (i.e. in the space occupied by the herbs in the container) the five Dhyani or Meditational Buddhas and their consorts.

The process of generating the Five Dhyani Buddhas in the container is as follows:

- After performing purification of the environment, visualize the Five Dhyani Buddhas appearing from emptiness in the container. In the center of the mandala is a white Vairocana and his consort; they appear from the seed-syllables OM and MUM. A blue Vajrasattva and is consort, located in the East, emerge from the seed-syllables HUM and LAM respectively. A yellow Ratnasambhava and his consort are in the South and they emerge respectively from the seed-syllables TRAM and MAM. In the West is a red Amitabha and his consort, who emerge from the seed-syllables AH and TAM. Located at the crowns, throats and hearts of each of these deities are the three universal syllables OM, AH and HUM. Light radiates from these three syllables and invokes the blessings and grace of the five real Dhyani Buddhas, who then merge with the five imaginal ones.
- From the fusion of the masculine and feminine energies of the deities and their consorts, red and white seminal fluids of bliss are visualized flowing down into the containers of herbs, transforming the herbs into the nectar of immortality and good health.
- Then, from the heart of the physician in the form of Vajrapani, rays of light are generated out to the five Dhyani Buddhas and their consorts, invoking them to generate incredible healing rays of light in the form of Dakinis — goddesses of offering. These offering goddesses please and seek the blessings and inspirations of all enlightened beings, Bodhisattvas and other celestial

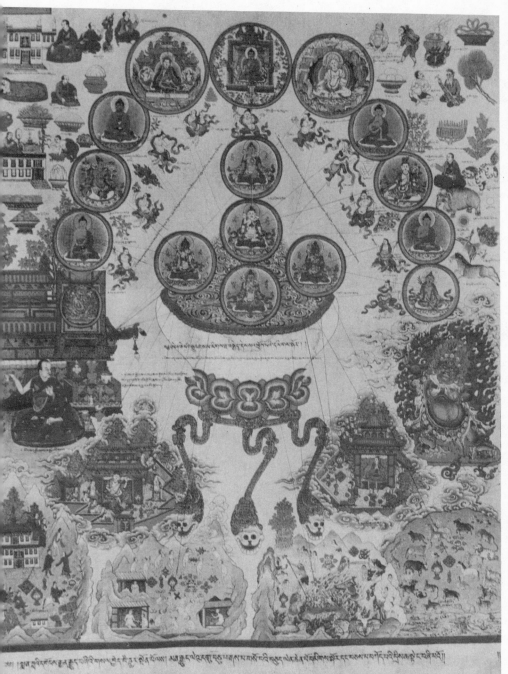

entities. They transmit their healing powers into the herbs in the container.

The light rays gather together the healing essence of all plants, minerals, and energies in the universe and transmit them into the herbs in container. These include the yellow luster of the fire element, the blue luster of the water element, the green luster of the wood and air elements, and the white luster of the metal or iron element. Each one is accompanied by the recitation of the mantra of the Buddha of the corresponding color as well as the exilers from the realms of the gods, demi-gods, human beings, animals and other beings.

- In a state of total calm and concentration, the rejuvenation mantra is now recited as follows: "Vairochana OM, Vajrasattva HUM, Ratnasambhava TAM, Amitabha HRI, Karmavajra AH." Recite this as many times as possible (traditionally, it should be recited 50,000 times). The nectar herb should be taken on an empty stomach, beginning at dawn on the first day of the waxing moon.
- Dissolve all the images and visualizations.
- Meditate on emptiness.
- Finish with the dedication and thanksgiving.

11
SELF-HEALING THROUGH THE
MEDICINE BUDDHA PRACTICE

INTRODUCTION

The power of healing through the practice of the Medicine Buddha visualization and meditation is deeply rooted in the Buddhist tradition and is a living and dynamic part of Tibetan Buddhism. There are many components in the practice which make it meaningful and transformative: self-confidence, positive thinking, faith, motivation, concentration, and reality orientation. But the most important component for the healing process is the ability to use and develop the power of creative imagination. This, in fact, is the crux of all advanced Buddhist practice.

In practicing self-healing, the Buddhist tradition identifies two related criteria:

1. confidence and self-esteem, and
2. the mental ability and courage to create a new self-image by transforming the harmful energy of psychological complexes and negativities into the beneficial energy of positive and inspiring mental images and symbols.

The basic psychological and healing principles that govern the Medicine Buddha self-healing practice are explained here. Anyone with the appropriate motivation may engage in it; however, in order to practice the advanced form of the Medicine Buddha a complete initiation from a qualified teacher is required.

PRELIMINARY STEPS

These steps are designed to help you prepare physically, mentally and spiritually to engage in the actual practice.

The first step is to insure that you are physically and mentally relaxed and in tune with your mind and body. This is accomplished by doing breathing exercises such as the ones mentioned in the book *Beyond the Relaxation Response* by Dr. Benson. While doing them, you might also want to keep wet towels handy to wipe your face, as well as have scented herbs nearby to help prevent drowsiness and dullness.

The second step is to become aware of your emotional state. If you notice feelings of anger or desire or, possibly, even of mental distraction or stagnation, try to get in touch with your emotion and identify its character. Once you know how you're feeling, use the following guide to select an appropriate focus for meditation and begin immediately.

- Excessive desire: Meditate on change and impermanence

- Anger and aggression: Meditate on love and patience

- Pride and self-importance: Meditate on parts of your body, such as the organs, one by one

- Confusion and bewilderment: Meditate on the causative factors in the past that lead to your current situation and how your present activities might affect your future experiences

- Distraction and discursiveness: Meditate on the breath by counting your inhalations and exhalations

Do not expend too much energy on these two preliminary steps. Use no more than a quarter of your practice time on these exercises.

The next step clearly establishes in the psyche the heightened level of motivation that is needed for the actual practice.

By understanding a fuller range of purposes for engaging in the self-healing practice, we can greatly increase our initial level of motivation. Broadly speaking, there are three levels of purpose for self-healing. These are to heal:

- a personal physical illness
- a personal psychological illness
- all illnesses in the world, including yours

Begin at the first level by accepting the need to heal your own physical illness. Now extend this image to include the healing of your psyche. Eventually, expand your purpose by imagining the ultimate healing of all that is sick and suffering in the world. By generating the need to free everything from pain and suffering, by making the whole universe free, one's own healing process will also progress. It will be nourished by the image of universal health.

The final step is to intensify this image of universal health by internally personifying it and seeking a relationship with this ideal person. This ideal universal healer is identified as the Medicine Buddha. The process of beginning the relationship occurs by imaging the ideal healer two feet in front of you (see illustration). The ideal healer should be imagined as alive and vibrant while you respectfully ask permission to have a healing relationship. The ideal healer responds warmly with the spirit of friendship and the bond is now established.

THE MEDICINE BUDDHA PRACTICE

The practitioner begins by visualizing rays of white light emanating in all directions from the heart of the Medicine Buddha; all enlightened beings and healers are extremely pleased. They in turn send healing rays back to the Medicine Buddha, who is now vibrating with extraordinary healing power and energy. From his heart, laser-like rays of blue light shoot towards the practitioner, who absorbs the healing light into his being as he inhales. The blue rays of light purify all the toxins and negativities, destroying them and congealing them into atoms of black smoke that are expelled as the practitioner exhales. The black smoke then disappears into the ground. This complete visualization sequence may be done three or more times.

The visualization sequence is now repeated, but the recipients of the healing are now imagined to be all the sick and suffering beings of the world.

Healing powers and energies have now been acquired from the Medicine Buddha in front of you, and you are now endowed with the qualities to carry out self-healing. Use this opportunity to empower the herbs, medications, or food items selected to aid your healing. Place these substances in a clean bowl in front of you and recite the Medicine Buddha Healing Mantra:

THAYATHA OM BEKAZAI BEKAZAI MAHA BEKAZAI RANZE SAMUGATHE SO HA

Repeat this mantra as many times as possible while visualizing the energy of the mantra empowering the substances with extraordinary healing powers.

When the recitation is complete, generate a sense of calmness and quietude in order to experience the healing and the joy which follows it. In a state of satisfaction, dissolve the image of the Medicine Buddha that has been in front of you. Finally, in a state of emptiness, dedicate all the merit you may have gained during this event to the entire universe and be thankful for this precious opportunity to heal.

12
THE TIBETAN
HEALTH HOROSCOPE

INTRODUCTION

Tibetan Buddhist astrology is a combination of both the Hindu and Chinese astrological systems in which it is assumed that the configuration of celestial bodies has a powerful influence over the individual and his health. The complexity of this subject is greatly reduced in this chapter by introducing the Tibetan Health Horoscope, which allows you to determine such influences. A knowledge of your year of birth is all that is needed to find your zodiacal sign in the chart below. Then, by the relationship between your sign and the days of the week, another chart enables you to determine when you will be most deeply affected by harmonious or inharmonious movements of the energy in the body.

This Tibetan Health Horoscope is recommended for:

- anyone interested in how astrology influences your life and energy activities

- anyone interested in health, and especially in the state and condition of your energy and chakras during particular days of the week

- healers, acupuncturists, massage therapists, and counselors, in order to decide which days of the week are best to work with their clients, when to decide on a major form of treatment, determine the balance of the energies, meridians and chakras in the body of the client on specific days of the week, and also to help guide the client about his treatment and behavior

- spiritual and religious practitioners, in order to determine when they should start a practice, a retreat, or a major spiritual commitment

FINDING YOUR ZODIAC SIGN

Years of Birth and Corresponding Zodiacal Signs

Hare	1903	1915	1927	1939	1951	1963
Dragon	1904	1916	1928	1940	1952	1964
Snake	1905	1917	1929	1941	1953	1965
Horse	1906	1918	1930	1942	1954	1966
Sheep	1907	1919	1931	1943	1955	1967
Monkey	1908	1920	1932	1944	1956	1968
Bird	1909	1921	1933	1945	1957	1969
Dog	1910	1922	1934	1946	1958	1970
Pig	1911	1923	1935	1947	1959	1971
Rat	1912	1924	1936	1948	1960	1972
Ox	1913	1925	1937	1949	1961	1973
Tiger	1914	1926	1938	1950	1962	1974

HOW TO USE THE HOROSCOPE

After having found your zodiac sign by checking the birth year chart, you can use the horoscope chart below to plan different kinds of activities according to which day of the week is best for the purpose. There are three types of days: favorable, friendly and antagonistic.

Favorable Days

For each zodiac sign, there are days of the week when the astral and elemental combinations are in optimal harmony and therefore extremely favorable and lucky. During these days the energy flow in the body and the chakras is also in its optimal state of balance and health for the week. As a result, this is the appropriate time to engage in any major health activities as well as undergo any forms of treatment aimed at further improving your energy flow, such as massage, acupuncture, moxibustion, meditation, and other energy-related therapies. This is also the time when you should undergo any major radical treatment such as chemotherapy or surgery, since the energy in your body is more active and healing as compared to the other days. In addition, since the astral and elemental combinations are extremely favorable for you, these are the days when you should choose to:

- make important decisions such as starting a new venture, buying a new house, moving to a new city, etc.

- start new relationships, meet important people, make decisions affecting your family and loved ones

- travel on important business or long holidays

- begin life-changing activities such as a spiritual practice, a diet plan, or exercise program

Friendly Days

These are the days when the astral and elemental combinations are good, and should be used as second choice or in case of emergencies for all the activities described above under favorable days.

Antagonistic Days

During these days of the week, the astral influences and elemental combinations are in total conflict and disharmony with you. It would be extremely unfavorable and unlucky for you to initiate or carry out any of the activities mentioned above. In case you are forced to carry out such activities on these days, there are specific prescriptions recommended in the Tibetan astrological literature which will prevent the negative and unlucky influences from affecting you and your activities. These prescriptions involve special meditations and prayers performed on your behalf, carrying out social service in your area, assisting needy people and obtaining special teachings or initiations.

THE HOROSCOPE CHART

Sign	Favorable	Friendly	Antagonistic
Rat	Wednesday	Tuesday	Saturday
Ox	Saturday	Wednesday	Thursday
Tiger	Thursday	Saturday	Friday
Hare	Thursday	Saturday	Friday
Dragon	Sunday	Wednesday	Thursday
Snake	Tuesday	Friday	Wednesday
Horse	Tuesday	Friday	Wednesday
Sheep	Friday	Monday	Thursday
Monkey	Friday	Thursday	Tuesday
Bird	Friday	Thursday	Tuesday
Dog	Monday	Wednesday	Thursday
Pig	Wednesday	Tuesday	Saturday

BIBLIOGRAPHY

Badmajew, P. and V. Badmajew, and L. Park. *Healing Herbs: The Heart of Tibetan Medicine*. Berkeley, CA: Red Lotus Press, 1982.

Benson, Dr. Herbert. *Beyond the Relaxation Response*. New York, New York: Berkley Books, 1985.

Chogyam, Ngakpa. *Rainbow of Liberated Energy*. Dorset, England: Element Books Ltd., 1986.

Clifford, Terry. *Tibetan Buddhist Medicine and Psychiatry, The Diamond Healing*. York Beach, ME: Samual Weiser, Inc., 1984.

Donden, Dr. Yeshi. *Health Through Balance*. Ithaca, New York. Snow Lion Publications, 1986.

Finckh, Dr. Elisabeth. *Foundations of Tibetan Medicine, Vol. I and Vol. II*. Somerset, England: Watkins and Robinson Books Ltd., 1978.

Finckh, Dr. Elisabeth. *Studies in Tibetan Medicine*. Ithaca, New York: Snow Lion Publications, 1988.

Mind and Mental Health in Tibetan Medicine. New York, New York. Potala Publications, 1988.

Norbu, Dawa (editor). *An Introduction to Tibetan Medicine*. New Delhi, India: Tibetan Review Publication, 1976.

Rapgay, Dr. Lobsang. *Tibetan Therapeutic Massage*. Dharamsala, India: Rapgay Publication, 1985.

Rapgay, Dr. Lobsang. *Tibetan Medicine: A Holistic Approach to Better Health*. Dharamsala, India: Rapgay Publication, 1985.

Rapgay, Dr. Lobsang. *The Art of Tibetan Medical Urinalysis*. Dharamsala, India: Rapgay Publication, 1986.

Rinpoche, Ven. Rechung. *Tibetan Medicine*. Berkeley, California: University of California Press, 1973.

Tibetan Medicine, Series No. 1 thru 9 and Series No. 2, Vol. II. Dharamsala, India: LTWA.

Tsarong, T. J., editor. *Fundamentals of Tibetan Medicine.* Dharamsala, India: Tibetan Medical Centre Publication, 1981.

Tsarong, T. J., editor. *Handbook of Traditional Tibetan Drugs.* Dharamsala, India: Tibetan Medical Centre Publication, 1986.

Index

A
adipose tissues 33
alchemy 127
allum staivum 130
angelica 128
anger 17, 18, 48, 56, 101, 107,
  142, 146, 163, 164, 169, 170,
  188
aniseed 128
anxiety 48, 106, 107, 110, 115,
  119, 131, 132
appetite loss 107, 123; poor 34
aquilaria 18 131
aquilaria 35 131
aquilaria agollocha 130
arthritis 119, 123
asafoetida 128
ashwagandha 128
asparagus racemosis root 128
Astanga Hrdaya 12
Ayurveda 11–13, 119, 127

B
Bagan 12, 24, 29–34, 37, 41, 42,
  44, 45, 63, 65, 67, 70, 73, 75,
  81, 91–98, 107, 116, 121, 123,
  125, 132, 176, 178
black pepper 128
blood 27, 33, 36, 55, 56, 62, 91,
  114, 119, 121, 123, 124, 130,
  173–176; detoxification 119,
  123
body temperature, low 31, 34
bones 33, 42
bowel movements, suppressed
  105

breath, shortness of 104
breathing problems 104; suppressed 104
Buddha 11, 12, 148, 157, 167,
  177, 180–182, 185, 187, 189,
  190

C
Caraka Samhita 12
cardamom 129
chest 33, 41, 84, 90, 95, 96, 104,
  112, 131; pains in upper 104
chills 31, 33, 130, 131
cinnamon 129
circulation, poor 33, 41, 42, 129
clarity 103, 121, 143, 146, 147,
  150, 152, 164
clove seeds 129
colds 104, 123, 129, 130, 131
colon 18, 29, 33
commitment 151, 173, 180, 192
compassion 11, 13, 117, 141,
  166, 170
complexion, pale 34
compulsiveness 106
congestion 104, 128, 129, 130
connecting to the Divine 151
constipation 31, 33, 40, 48, 71,
  72, 105, 106, 128
convulsions 104
coriander 129
coughs 123, 129, 130
cucumber seeds 129
cumin seeds 129

D
dandelion root 129
dedication 44, 151, 152, 185
diarrhea 25, 31, 34, 48, 72, 107,
  129, 130
digestion, difficulty in 104;
  poor 24, 48, 107; slow 34

BIODATA

Lopsang Rapgay, is a Tibetan Buddhist monk trained as a physician in the Tibetan tradition of medicine. He is currently completing his training as a clinical psychologist and practices in West Los Angeles. He has written several books on Mind, Body Medicine and Healing.

He may be contacted at: 2206 Benecia Avenue, West Los Angeles, CA 90064

BOOKS OF RELATED INTEREST

The Astrology of the Seers
A Guide to Vedic Astrology by David Frawley
    ISBN 1-878423-05-3   342 pp. $18.95

Ayurvedic Healing
A Comprehensive Guide by David Frawley
    ISBN 1-878423-00-2   388 pp. $18.95

From the River of Heaven
Hindu and Vedic Knowledge for the Modern Age by David Frawley
    ISBN 1-878423-01-1   180 pp. $12.95

Gods, Sages and Kings
Vedic Secrets of Ancient Civilization by David Frawley
    ISBN 1-878423-08-8   396 pp. $19.95

Wisdom of the Ancient Seers
Mantras of the *Rig Veda* by David Frawley
    ISBN 1-878423-16-9   260 pp. $14.95

Tantric Yoga and the Wisdom Goddesses
Spiritual Secrets of Ayurveda by David Frawley
    ISBN 1-878423-17-7   256 pp. $16.95

Fundamentals of Vedic Astrology
Vedic Astrologer's Handbook, Volume I by Bepin Behari
    ISBN 1-878423-09-6   280 pp. $14.95

Planets in the Signs and Houses
Vedic Astrologer's Handbook, Volume II by Bepin Behari
    ISBN 1-878423-10-X   258 pp. $14.95

The Oracle of Rama
by David Frawley
    ISBN 1-878423-19-3   208 pp. $12.95

Astrological Healing Gems by Shivaji Bhattacharjee
    ISBN 1-878423-07-X   128 pp. $7.95

Natural Healing Through Ayurveda
by Dr. Subhash Ranade
    ISBN 1-878423-13-4   195 pp. $14.95

Interacting With Society
Life Strategies Series by Edward F. Tarabilda
    ISBN 1-878423-03-7   176 pp. $7.95

Happy, Healthful Longevity
Life Strategies Series by Edward F. Tarabilda
    ISBN 1-878423-02-9   160 pp. $7.95

The Spiritual Quest
Life Strategies Series by Edward F. Tarabilda
    ISBN 1-87842 3-04-5   125 pp. $7.95

VEDIC ASTROLOGY COMPUTER PROGRAM

PC-JYOTISH, a Vedic (Hindu) astrology computer program for IBM compatable computers, is now available. Its features include:

- *South & North India chart styles*
- Rasi (sign) and Bhava (house) charts
- *Navamsa and other Varga (divisional) charts*
- *Shadbala*
- *Summary Tables — relationships & locations; Sign/house qualities & relationships*
- *Nakshatras — lords/sublords & pada lords*
- *Vimshopak*
- *Planetary Significators*
- *Ashtaka Varga — complete*
- *Vimshottari dashas, bhuktis & sub-bhuktis (365¼ or 360 day year)*
- *Pop-up Transit window with Ashtaka Varga & Nakshatra divisions*
- *Aspects Table*
- *Range of Ayanamshas or your own*
- *Easy to use, user driven program*
- *Mouse support*
- *Changing input data immediately alters on-screen tables & charts*
- *Pull-down menus*
- *Print to file or any ASCII printer*
- *Complete on-screen functions*
- *As many charts & tables on-screen as user desires*
- *User arranges windows on-screen*
- *Chart storage limited only by disk space*
- *Manual with glossary by David Frawley*
- *Program range: 1500 BC to 2200 AD*
- *Requires 420k ram*
- *Color/mono, hi-res mode — no graphics card required*
- *The Outer Planets, and more*

DEMO program $5.00 (refunded if program purchased) plus s/h.

For more information call or write:

Passage Press
P.O. Box 21713
Salt Lake City, UT 84121-0713
(801) 942–1440